CARDIO-THORACIC SURGERY

WHAT IS NEW IN CURRENT PRACTICE

CARDIO-THORACIC SURGERY

WHAT IS NEW IN CURRENT PRACTICE

Proceedings of the Second International Symposium,
Bad Oeynhausen, 5-7 September 1991

Editors:

K. MINAMI
R. KÖRFER
J. WADA

 1992

EXCERPTA MEDICA
AMSTERDAM – LONDON – NEW YORK – TOKYO

International Congress Series No. 985
ISBN 0 444 89267 2

This book is printed on acid-free paper.

Published by:
Elsevier Science Publishers B.V.
P.O. Box 211
1000 AE Amsterdam
The Netherlands

Library of Congress Cataloging-in-Publication Data

Cardio-thoracic surgery : what is new in current practice : proceedings of the second international
    symposium, Bad Oeynhausen, 5-7 September 1991 / editors, K. Minami, R. Körfer, J. Wada.
      p. cm. -- (International congress series : no. 985)
    Includes index.
    ISBN 0-444-89267-2 (alk. paper)
    1. Heart--Surgery--Congresses. 2. Chest--Surgery--Congresses.
    I. Minami, K. II. Körfer, Reiner. III. Wada, Jurō, 1922- .
    IV. Series.
    [DNLM: 1. Heart Surgery--methods--congresses.   W3 EX89 no. 985]
    RD598.C3537   1992
    617.4'12059--dc20
    DNLM/DLC
    for Library of Congress   92-9994
                                                    CIP

In order to ensure rapid publication this volume was prepared using a method of electronic text processing known as Optical Character Recognition (OCR). Scientific accuracy and consistency of style were handled by the author. Time did not allow for the usual extensive editing process of the Publisher.

Printed in The Netherlands.

PREFACE

The second Symposium on Cardio-Thoracic Surgery held in Bad Oeynhausen September 5-7, 1991 was placed under the very evocative theme: "What's new in current practice" and covered a very large spectrum with the newest approaches in each aspect of cardio vascular surgery.

After the opening remarks from the President R. KÖRFER, the Minister of Health H. HEINEMANN, the Dean K. HINRIKHSEN, J. WADA President of the International Society of Cardio-Thoracic Surgeons, and P. SATTER President of the German Society for Thoracic and Cardio-Vascular Surgery, the first session was devoted to three main topics of congenital surgery: palliation or correction of complex lesions (Y. KAWASHIMA), total cavo pulmonary connection (T. EBELS), and arterial switch operation (H. MEISNER).

In the second session the still crucial and unsettled question of myocardial preservation was treated by two famous pioneers in that field, M. BRAIMBRIGE and H. BRETSCHNEIDER with a presentation on trauma metabolism and the heart by K. VYSKA.

Pulsatile and non pulsatile flow in extra corporeal circulation were compared by an expert on this subject: K. TAYLOR and by K. MINAMI.

Everybody now agrees to reduction of the blood use in open heart surgery and this topic was well documented by the presentations of E. WOLNER, JP. GARDAZ and R. KÖRFER.

In session V the increasing role of Doppler echocardiography before and during cardiac surgery was emphasized by S. MIHAILEANU in valve reconstruction, N. NANDA in the assessment of initial regurgitation, S. TAKAMOTO in aortic dissection and H. MEYER in congential heart diseases.

New trends in valve surgery were exposed by the best experts in the field C. DURAN (reconstruction of cardiac valves), W. ANGELL (stentless bioprosthesis), A. DZIATKOWIAK (homograft) and P. BRUKE (homograft bank).

Session VII on surgical treatment of malignant tachyarrhythmias, was specially expected with such pioneers as my friend, and for a long time, companion G. GUIRAUDON (ventricular tachyarrhythmias), T. IWA (WPW syndrome), V. DOR (ventricular arrhythmias after myocardial infarction or aneurysm) and the use of implantable defibrillators by G. ALMASSI.

I had the great honor to chair also the last session on the current state of heart/heart lung transplantation with the newest therapeutic refinements reported by the prestigious Stanford Group (V. STARNES and N. SHUMWAY) the impressive series of M. YACOUB and the long term immunological insults on the coronary arteries of the heart and the bronchi of the lungs.

A short final discussion with Y. NOSE, P. WALTER and F. HUGER on indications of congenital and valvular surgery, ventricular assist devices and quality of life after heart surgery concluded this largely attended meeting, moderated by

such outstanding colleagues as F. SEBENING, H. HUYSMANS, L. LACQUET, R. OMOTO, C. OLIN, D. SCHULTE, N. ALTHAUS and illustrated by an exposition of more than 30 posters, and a visit in the very active cardio vascular center of our hosts who organized so well this most enjoyable and successful symposium.
Looking forward for the third one soon!

C. CABROL
Sce de Chirurgie Cardio-Vasculaire - Hôpital LA PITIE - PARIS - FRANCE

CONTENTS

© 1992 Elsevier Science Publishers B.V. All rights reserved
Cardio-thoracic surgery. K. Minami et al. editors.

Surgical treatment of complex congenital heart disease in neonates and infancy – palliative or corrective procedure

Yasunaru Kawashima[1], Hikaru Matsuda[2], Toshikatu Yagihara[1], Yasuhisa Simazaki[2], Kyoichi Nishigaki[1], Masahiko Iio[2], Yoshio Aragaki[3] and Tetsuo Kamiya[3]

[1]Department of Cardiovascular Surgery, National Cardiovascular Center, Fujishirodai 5-7-1, Suita, Akaka 565, Japan, [2]First Department of Surgery, Osaka University Hospital, Fukushima 1-1-50, Fukushima-ku, Osaka 553, Japan, and [3]Department of Pediatrics, National Cardiovascular Center, Fujisirodai 5-7-1, Suita, Osaka 565, Japan

Introduction

The current trend in pediatric cardiac surgery is towards the very young. It is generally considered that primary repair as early as possible is far better than a two-stage operation. However, there are two conditions governing the recommendation of primary repair in neonates and infancy. First, the risk of primary repair in infancy should be lower than or at least the same as that of the two-stage operation, including the risk of two operations and the risk while waiting for the second operation. Second, the late results of primary repair should be better or at least not worse than that of the two-stage operation. However, conclusions on this matter based on clinical follow-up studies are lacking or scanty.

In this paper, we would like to present some of the data on this matter obtained from experiences in Osaka University Hospital (OUH) and in the National Cardiovascular Center (NCVC).

Definitions

The subjects of this paper are confined to certain types of complex congenital cardiac anomalies in neonates and infancy. In this study, complex cardiac anomalies were classified into 4 groups from the viewpoint of the surgical program.

Group 1: patients who undergo definite palliation and for whom corrective surgery is not indicated.

Group 2: patients who usually undergo correction without palliation in neonates and infancy. They include total anomalous pulmonary venous connection (TAPVC), transposition of the great arteries (TGA) without left ventricular outflow tract obstruction (LVOTO), truncus, etc.

Group 3: patients who usually undergo the two-stage operation, the first-stage operation as neonates or in infancy. They include tetralogy of Fallot (TF) with pulmonary atresia (PA) and major aortopulmonary collateral artery (MAPCA), hypoplastic left heart syndrome (HLHS), etc.

2

Group 4: this group of patients is the subject of the present study. They include interruption of the aortic arch (IAA) and coarctation of the aorta (CoA) with other cardiac anomaly, TF, and common atrioventricular canal, (CAVC), etc. The selection of one-stage or two-stage correction is still controversial for these groups of patients.

Palliative procedures indicated for these anomalies are numerous and they were classified into 3 groups according to their aims. The first group of palliative procedures is the classical and the purpose of these procedures is purely to improve the patient's condition. The second group is aimed to prepare for the second-stage procedure, which is usually corrective. The third group of procedures is not actual palliation but partial correction of the combination of anomalies.

Patients, operations and results

The following three groups of patients were studied.

Interruption of the aortic arch (IAA) and coarctation of the aorta (CoA) associated with other cardiac anomalies

Since 1978 in NCVC 32 patients with IAA and 46 patients with CoA associated with other cardiac anomalies were operated upon. All of the former and 44 (96%) of the latter were operated upon as neonates or in infancy either with palliative or with corrective procedures. Initially, two-stage operations were performed. However, one-stage repair has been preferred to two-stage repair since 1989.

The results of these operations are shown in Fig. 1. Previously, the results of

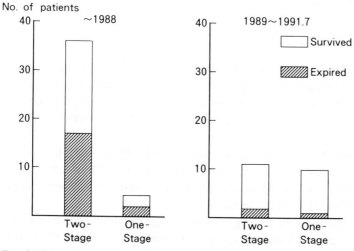

Fig. 1. The result of operation for IAA and CoA with cardiac anomalies in patients operated upon in NCVC.

two-stage correction in neonates and infants were quite unsatisfactory. This has improved recently. The operative mortality of one-stage correction since 1989 was 10% and was not significantly different from that of two-stage correction, which was 18%.

Tetralogy of Fallot (TF)

For more than 10 years it had been our program to correct this anomaly at 1 or 2 yr of age when patients reached a weight of more than 8 kg [1]. Following this program, 82 patients of 1 or 2 yr of age underwent corrective surgery in OUH and 138 patients in NCVC between 1978 and 1990. One of the former and 6 of the latter expired within 30 days of operation resulting in an overall mortality of 3.2%.

During the same period, the pediatric cardiology department of NCVC accepted 184 newborns and infants with this anomaly. These patients were treated according to the above-mentioned program. Most of them had already been operated on and some of them reached 2 yr of age before surgery for various reasons. Eight patients expired before surgery and 3 died related to palliative surgery, which had been performed in 35 patients. Thus, altogether 11 out of 184 patients expired before corrective surgery or reaching 2 yr of age, resulting in total mortality of 6.0%.

Therefore, the overall cumulative mortality of the patients who underwent the surgical program of correcting tetralogy of Fallot at age 1 or 2 yr is estimated to be 9% as a result of the following calculations.

Non-surgical and palliative surgical mortality = 6.0%

Corrective surgical mortality = 3.2%

$$\text{Overall mortality} = 6.0 + (100 - 6.0) \times \frac{3.2}{100}$$

$$= 9.0\%$$

Common atrioventricular canal (CAVC)

Between 1978 and 1990, 5 patients aged 1 or 2 yr with CAVC underwent repair without death in OUH and 26 patients aged 1 or 2 yr with one death in NCVC. Total mortality for this series of 31 patients was thus 3.2%. It has been our method of operation to utilize the endocardial cushion prosthesis reported previously to compensate the deficient endocardial cushion [2].

During the same period, 39 patients with CAVC visited NCVC as neonates and during infancy. Two of them underwent pulmonary artery manipulation without death. Thirty-seven patients were medically treated until they were older than 1 yr and underwent corrective surgery, or reached 2 yrs of age without surgery for various reasons. Ten patients expired during this period, resulting in a mortality of 27%. Thus the patients who followed the present program of treatment had a cumulative non-surgical and palliative surgical mortality of 25.6% (10/39).

Thus the overall mortality in patients who underwent the surgical program of correcting CAVC at age 1 or 2 yr was 28% according to the following calculations.

Non-surgical and palliative surgical mortality = 25.6%

Corrective surgical mortality = 3.2%

$$\text{Overall mortality} = 25.6 + (100 - 25.6) \times \frac{3.2}{100}$$

$$= 28.0$$

Discussion

The results of surgical and non-surgical treatments for 3 kinds of rather common complex cardiac anomalies are presented, following our present treatment programs. Based on these data, we would like to discuss whether we should keep these programs or modify them. The major question is whether we should perform corrective surgery for these anomalies during the neonatal period and infancy.

Interruption of the aortic arch and coarctation of the aorta associated with other cardiac anomalies

Although our routine program of operating on these abnormalities has changed from two-stage correction to one-stage correction, we still utilized two-stage correction even after 1989. There is obviously the tendency that the patients who underwent two-stage correction had more complicated cardiac anomalies than those who underwent one-stage correction. Therefore, there is a possibility that if we apply the one-stage operation to all these patients regardless of the associated cardiac anomalies, the result of surgery may be worsened because of technical difficulties and prolonged cardiac arrest. From the data presented in this paper, it is not possible to speculate on the exact outcome of the program treating all these abnormalities with a one-stage operation. However, the data from other reports [3] and also from our initial experiences are encouraging for one-stage repair.

Tetralogy of Fallot

As reported above, overall cumulative mortality for patients having corrective surgery at 1 or 2 yr of age was as high as 9%. As our present mortality of corrective surgery at this age is about 1-2%, overall mortality may be a little less at the present time and will be about 7%. Should we then operate on these patients correctively during the neonatal period and infancy when corrective surgical mortality is less than 7%? There is a good possibility that the operative mortality could be kept less than 7% even though we operate on them when neonates or infants. However, we should also consider the late results of the patients who underwent correction in such an early life. The late results should be the same as or better than those of the patients who underwent correction at age 1 or 2 yrs.

However, comparative study of late results between the patients who underwent correction at age 1 or 2 yr and those at less than 1 yr is not possible as data on the latter group of patients are lacking. We have to estimate the long-term results of these patients by some means.

As we have previously reported [4,5], significant pulmonary regurgitation after correction affects the late hemodynamic results. On the other hand, significant pulmonary regurgitation was found in 66% of patients who were operated upon with the use of pulmonary transannular patch, but only in 22% of patients without transannular patch [6]. As we have reported previously, it is our method to correct tetralogy without or with minimum right ventriculotomy, and the use of transannular patch is limited to less than 50% of cases.

Do we more often incise the pulmonary valve ring when we correct tetralogy of Fallot in neonates and infants? So far no answer is available but from our limited experience, the pulmonary valve ring of the infant seems to be more distensible than that of older children and, therefore, the answer is very likely to be 'no'.

Another question arises whether the pulmonary valve ring grows with age after correction. The answer is suggested to be positive for patients without transannular patch but for patients with transannular patch, it is suggested to depend on the compensatory growth of the native valve ring tissue. This was studied in 15 patients who underwent repair without transannular patch and in 15 patients with transannular patch. The pulmonary valve rings grew with age and there were no differences between the two groups. Details of this study will be reported separately [7]. The results of this study indicate that no particularly frequent development of pulmonary valve restenosis will be anticipated to develop even after correction in neonates and infants.

As a conclusion of these considerations, it is most likely that no particularly significant drawback in the late post-operative period will be found even though patients with tetralogy of Fallot undergo the corrective surgery as neonates or infants. We may recommend operating on this anomaly correctively in neonates and infants if the operative mortality could be kept below 7% on condition that no patient expires before having corrective surgery.

Common atrioventricular canal

The overall cumulative mortality for the patients with CAVC who underwent corrective surgery at 1 or 2 yr of age was as high as 28%, as so many patients expire before undergoing surgery. On the other hand, mortality from corrective surgery was as low as 3% if patients were operated upon at age 1 or 2 yr. From these data, it is obvious that the corrective surgery is recommendable for this anomaly in neonates and infants as we could presume that the result of correction in the first year of life will be a mortality of less than 28%. This is on condition that the late results of patients who underwent correction before 1 yr of age are the same or even better than those of patients corrected at age 1 or 2. Although the number of corrective operations before 1 yr of age is quite limited up to now, so far we have corrected 13 patients in OUH, with 2 deaths, resulting in a mortality rate of 15%.

For the correction of CAVC, the use of septal patches, which have no potential to grow, is unavoidable. The sequelae due to the presence of this patch should be considered particularly when patients are operated upon in the neonatal period and infancy as the material does not grow and approximately one-third of the circumference of the A-V valve is usually replaced with this material after the correction.

If the mitral valve ring, two-thirds of which has been replaced with prosthetic material at the age of 1 month, grows according to the normal growth pattern, it is roughly estimated to be the size of that of 7.5-yr-old child when the patient is 15 yr old. If the patient is operated upon with the same technique at age 2 yr, it will be the size of that of 9-yr-old child when the patient is 15 yr old. These sizes are a little too small for adult patients but it is reasonable to speculate that the other part of the atrioventricular valve circumference will grow and compensate the septal portion replaced with patch.

It should also be considered whether the presence of the septal patch has some influence on the development or progression of mitral and/or tricuspid regurgitations after long periods of time. Not only because of the limited circumference due to the septal patch, but also because of downward displacement of the attachment of septal leaflets the A-V valve regurgitation may develop after long periods of follow-up time. To avoid these phenomena, the authors have developed the so-called endocardial cushion prosthesis with two wings on both sides of the straight patch for the compensation of the septal leaflets of atrioventricular valves.

It is not clear whether this is the result of using endocardial cushion prosthesis or not, but the progression of the mitral valve regurgitation was quite rare among the patients who underwent repair with this technique, as shown in Fig. 2. From these data of medical and surgical treatment both during and after infancy, one-stage corrective surgery in neonates and infancy is now recommended, as the risk of one-stage operation in infancy is far below 28% in our experience. Although the use of endocardial cushion prosthesis seems to be preferable even for small

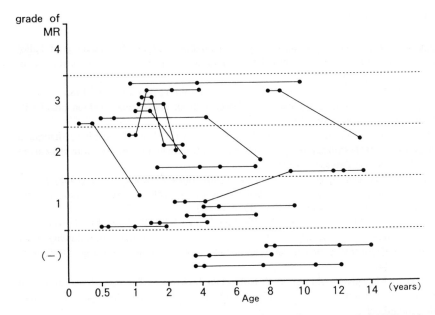

Fig. 2. Change of the intensity of mitral regurgitation after repair of CAVC with endocardial cushion prosthesis in patients operated upon in OUH.

babies to minimize the late sequelae, it should be evaluated in future as the atrioventricular valve leaflets in small babies are quite friable to suture to the wings of endocardial cushion prosthesis.

From the data we have presented in this paper, it seems that for both TF and CAVC, the one-stage correction in neonates and infancy is recommendable. However, the calculations and speculations we have presented were made on condition that no patient will expire before early one-stage correction. Among the non-surgically treated patients, one with TF and two with CAVC expired in the neonatal period. To salvage all these small patients, we have to operate on them very early in their lives.

Conclusion

One-stage corrective surgery in neonates and infancy is recommended (1) for interruption of the aortic arch and coarctation of the aorta associated with other cardiac anomalies, (2) for tetralogy of Fallot, if the risk is less than 7% and the use of transannular patch is less than 50%, and (3) for common atrioventricular canal, if the risk is less than 28%. It is actually far below that in our experience and therefore it is indicated. The use of endocardial cushion prosthesis is preferable. These conclusions are made on condition that no patient expires before reaching surgery when the new program is utilized.

8

References

1. Kawashima Y, Kitamura S, Yagihara T (1981) Corrective surgery for tetralogy of Fallot without or with minimal right ventriculotomy and with repair of the pulmonary valve. Circulation 64 (Suppl. 2): 147–153.
2. Kawashima Y, Matsuda H, Hirose H, Nakano S, Shimazaki Y, Miyamoto K (1983) Surgical treatment of complete atrioventricular canal defect with an endocardial cushion prosthesis. Circulation 68 (Suppl. 2): 139–143.
3. Yasui H, Kado H, Nakano E, Yonenaga K, Mitani A, Tomita Y, Iwao H, Yoshii K, Mizoguchi Y, Sunagawa H (1987) Primary repair of interrupted aortic arch and severe aortic stenosis in neonates. J Thorac Cardiovasc Surg 93: 539–545.
4. Kawashima Y, Matsuda H, Hirose H, Nakano S, Shirakura R, Kobayashi J (1985) Ninety consecutive corrective operations for tetralogy of Fallot with or without minimal right ventriculotomy. J Thorac Cardiovasc Surg 90: 856–863.
5. Bove EL, Byrum CJ, Thomas FD, Kavey RW, Sondheimer HM, Blackman MS, Parker FB Jr (1983) The influence of pulmonary insufficiency on right ventricular function following repair of tetralogy of Fallot. Evaluation using radio-nuclide ventriculography. J Thorac Cardiovasc Surg 85: 691–696.
6. Kawashima Y, Matsuda H, Shimazaki Y, Kobayashi J, Ikawa S. The role of transatrial and transpulmonary approach with no or minimum right ventriculotomy in the repair of tetralogy of Fallot. Submitted.
7. Iio M, Matsuda H, Kawashima Y, et al. In preparation.

Right atrial auricle as inter-caval tunnel in the total cavo-pulmonary connexion: method to avoid the sinus node and its blood supply

Tjark Ebels, Nynke J. Elzenga, Ursula Brenken, Johannes L. Bams, Jabik van Os and Anton Eijgelaar
Thorax Centre and Departments of Paediatric Cardiology and Anaesthesiology, University Hospital Groningen, The Netherlands

Introduction

The total cavo-pulmonary connexion, first described by Puga and associates [1], promises to be a viable alternative for the 'classic' Fontan operation [2,3], particularly in complex malformations involving left atrioventricular valve atresia or hypoplasia. Experimental work by DeLeval and colleagues has indicated that cavo-pulmonary connexions are associated with a lower resistance over the reconstruction than is the case in the 'classic' Fontan operation [2]. Additionally, the conduit in a 'classic' Fontan operation has the potential of becoming obstructed, leading to reoperation in 41% of the patients at 16 yr [4]. It remains uncertain, however, if the intra-atrial semi-synthetic tunnel employed in the total cavo-pulmonary connexion as described by DeLeval and Jonas can also be obstructed late after the operation. Furthermore, the suture line of this intra-atrial tunnel crosses the area of the sinus node or its blood supply, thus endangering perpetuation of sinus rhythm just as in the Mustard and Senning operations [5]. Arrhythmias have been reported in 22% of patients operated with the use of an intra-atrial synthetic tunnel, and even accounted for 40% of the mortality [6].

The aim of this paper is to describe a modified method for the total cavo-pulmonary connexion, employing the right auricle as an intra-atrial tunnel connecting the inferior to the superior caval vein, thus evading the area of the sinus node, and adding growth potential to the tunnel.

Material and Methods

Patients

From November 1988 until November 1990 we used the total cavo-pulmonary connexion in all 17 consecutive patients that were operated for any type of univentricular atrioventricular connexion at the University Hospital in Groningen. The right auricle was used in 12 patients as an intercaval tunnel carrying the inferior caval blood towards the superior caval vein. The diagnoses of these 12 patients are tabulated in Table 1. The right auricle was not used as an intercaval tunnel in 5 patients.

Reasons not to employ the right auricle were: redo Fontan procedures in two patients, in which the right auricle had been used in the previous operation. The right auricle was not used in a case of left atrial isomerism, because the morphologically left auricle was too small, thus a semi-synthetic tunnel was used. In two patients at the start of this series of cavo-pulmonary connexions the right auricle was not employed, because the risk to the sinus node was considered to be too great. Instead the atrial septal defect was simply closed, and no intra-atrial tunnel was used.

Operative procedure

All operations were done with the aid of cariopulmonary bypass and moderate hypothermia. Cold crystalloid cardioplegia was used in operative phases when the heart had to be opened. In all twelve patients the right superior caval vein was divided at the level of the right pulmonary artery. Cranial and caudal ends of the divided superior caval vein were then individually anastomosed to their respective aspects of the right pulmonary artery branch, creating as wide an anastomosis as

Table 1. Diagnoses and outcome of the 12 patients with a right auricular tunnel in the total cavopulmonary connexion

Pat. No.	Age (yr)	Diagnosis	Outcome
1	3.4	Tricuspid atresia, TGA	Alive
2	5.1	C-TGA, hypoplastic LV, azygos cont.	Alive
3	4.2	VSD, straddling tricuspid, hypopl.	Alive
4	3.9	Pulmonary atresia, intact VS	Alive
5	16.6	DILV, pulmonary atresia	Alive
6	4.0	Tricuspid atresia, concordant VAC	Alive
7	3.4	Tricuspid atresia, TGA	Alive
8	5.0	Dextrocardia, RAA, TAPVD, AVSD, bilat SCV's, hypopl. LV, disc. VAC, pulmonary atresia	Alive
9	2.3	Tricuspid atresia, concordant VAC	Alive
10	4.2	DORA, AVSD, DORV, hypopl. LV	Died, endocarditis
11	10.8	C-TGA, hypopl. systemic ventricle	Died, high PVR
12	3.8	VSD, straddling tricuspid, hypopl. RV, TGA	Alive

AVSD, atrioventricular septal defect; C-TGA, congenitally correct transposition of the great arteries; DILV, double inlet left ventricle; DORA, double outlet right atrium; DORV, double outlet right ventricle; hypopl., hypoplastic; LV, left ventricle; PVR, pulmonary vascular resistance; RAA, right atrial isomerism; RV, right ventricle; TGA, transposition of the great arteries; SCV, superior caval vein; VAC, ventriculo-arterial connexion; VS, ventricular septum; VSD, ventricular septal defect.

was possible. In the two patients with an additional left superior caval vein, this vein was also divided and the cranial end was anastomosed end-to-side to the left pulmonary artery; the caudal aspect of the left superior caval vein was closed. In the two patients with a right-sided heart the operation was performed in mirror image.

The operative photographs and clarifying drawings are of a patient with tricuspid atresia and a discordant ventriculo-arterial connexion. In order to prepare the right auricle for the tunnel an incision in the right atrium has to be

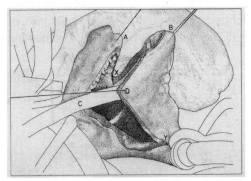

Fig. 1. The first incisions are made into the right auricle preparing it for construction of an intercaval tunnel. The first incision has a 'fish mouth' appearance, running in an antero-posterior direction on medial and lateral sides of the right auricle. On the lateral side the incision is carried to the terminal crest (C). On the left (medial) side the incision stops at the superior muscle bundle of the atrial septum (X). Cranial (A) and caudal (B) parts of the crescent of the right atrium are retracted by stay sutures. The atrial wall can be seen to be hypertrophied. The second incision is in the right lateral wall and runs from point C along the terminal crest to the level of the Eustachian valve of the inferior caval vein (Y). Thus a flap of right atrial wall is created, of which the right-angled cranio-posterior corner D is retracted by a stay suture. Points X and Y are the limits of the incision.

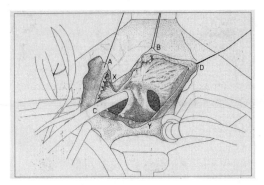

Fig. 2. The lateral atrial wall is retracted antero-inferiorly with a stay suture at point D, giving a panoramic insight into the right atrium, and the atrial septum can be inspected. The coronary sinus can be seen to be located inferiorly of the atrial septal defect, through which a sump drains the left atrium.

made in an antero-posterior fashion, caudal of the auricle. The posterior limit of the initial incision is the terminal crest, then an angle of 90° is made and the incision is continued in an inferior direction, along the terminal crest, until the level of the Eustachian valve is reached (Fig. 1).

The inferior part of the lateral atrial wall is retracted with a stay suture, giving a panoramic view of the atrial septum and defect (Fig. 2).

If an atrial septal defect does not exist, the oval fossa is excised. The usual abundance of muscle bars in the auricle is trimmed down, so as to create as smooth an inner surface of the tunnel as is possible.

The superior crescent of the right auricle is incised so as to create a quadrangular flap of atrial muscle (Fig. 3), which is then sutured to the anterior part of the junction of the inferior caval vein with the right atrium, usually a somewhat muscular Eustachian valve (Fig. 4).

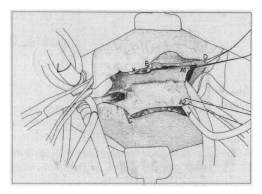

Fig. 3. A quadrangular flap of atrial muscle is created from the superior crescent of atrium, by a small incision along the top, splitting point A into A1 and A2. Points A1 and A2 are retracted caudally with stay sutures. Additionally, in this drawing, the superior caval vein is divided almost completely.

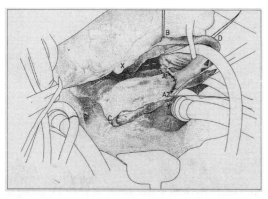

Fig. 4. The quadrangular flap of the right auricle is sutured along the posterior limit of the atrial septal defect starting at point X at the cranial end and from there to the entrance of the inferior caval vein into the atrium, where the flap is sutured to the Eustachian valve from point A1 to A2.

On the left side of the flap, the suture line courses via the right side of the coronary sinus orifice, the posterior rim of the atrial septal defect towards the superior aspect of the atrial septum. This leaves the coronary sinus draining into the pulmonary venous circulation. On the right side the auricle is sutured to the posterior aspect of the incision along the terminal crest (Fig. 5). Care must be taken to make the tunnel at least as wide as the inferior caval vein.

The cardiac end of the divided superior caval vein can be widened by a triangular flap of pericardium on the right lateral side. Preferably one should visualize the sinus node artery before this incision, so as to avoid damage to the sinus node blood supply. The flap of right atrial wall is then sutured down again, its posterior edge is sutured obliquely over the tunnel, and its superior edge is sutured to the cut edge of the auricle, adjacent to the atrioventricular groove, thus closing the atrium. All sutures are made with absorbable suture material (Fig. 6).

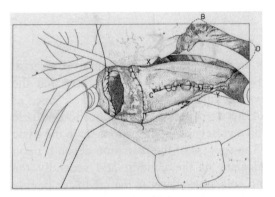

Fig. 5. The cranial end of the divided superior caval vein is anastomosed to the right pulmonary artery. The posterior part of the anastomosis is already sutured. The lateral suture line of the tunnel can be seen to run from point C to point Y.

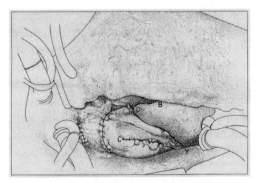

Fig. 6. Repair is completed by suturing the lateral atrial flap obliquely over the tunnel. To accomplish closure of the atrium, point D is sutured to point X, the suture line running from there anteriorly to point B. From the joined points D-X the suture line runs obliquely over the tunnel to the joined points A2-Y.

Results

Of the twelve patients operated with a right auricular tunnel two died (17%; CL: 6%-35%). One patient died due to a pulmonary vascular resistance of 3.4 Wood Units; additionally, a previous Blalock-Hanlon atrial septectomy made the tunnel encroach somewhat on the right upper pulmonary vein, thus leading to obstruction. The second patient died of endocarditis and subsequent stenosis of the superior cavopulmonary anastomosis. Some of the patients had temporary pleural or abdominal effusions necessitating drainage. All 10 survivors have been discharged in NYHA class I. No patient has had any late untoward effects of the operation such as protein-losing enteropathy. One patient who had initially been operated without the use of an intercaval intra-atrial tunnel was reoperated, because the wide right atrium proved to create a substantial resistance. One patient developed a sick sinus syndrome after the operation and subsequently received a pacemaker.

Comment

The late results of Fontan operations are only gradually beginning to emerge. From the combined Bordeaux and Birmingham study one can infer that the Fontan operation is not truly a curative operation because of a rising chance of reoperation after 10-15 yr [4]. Many of these reoperations are related to synthetic conduit obstruction, widely employed in a variety of modifications upon the basic principle of the Fontan operation [7]. The success of the palliation depends upon two aspects: firstly the unobstructed state of the conduit and secondly the perpetuation of sinus rhythm. Puga and colleagues deserve the credit for having had the imagination to find a simple solution for a difficult problem: the cavo-pulmonary connexion for atresia of the left-sided atrioventricular valve [1].

A cavo-pulmonary connexion enables a relatively lateral position of the intra-atrial patch, thus ensuring an unobstructed pulmonary venous blood flow. In contrast, for an atrio-pulmonary connexion the intra-atrial patch must be located far more medially, thus encroaching upon the channel from the left-sided pulmonary veins to the right-sided atrioventricular valve. The higher central venous pressure then makes the relatively medially located patch bulge to the left, thus further obstructing the pulmonary venous blood flow. An auriculo-pulmonary connexion probably has the same bad chance of pulmonary venous obstruction as has a connexion of the atrial roof with the pulmonary artery. It has been well documented that the presence of these large intra-atrial patches to divert pulmonary venous blood to the right-sided atrioventricular valve carries a poor prognosis [8].

Even with the hemodynamic 'atrial kick' caused by sinus rhythm the cardiac output of patients after a Fontan operation is subnormal. Absence of sinus rhythm lowers the cardiac output even further. Therefore, all operative procedures should be directed at avoidance of all conducting tissues, not only the atrioventricular node, but also the sinus node and its blood supply. The arrhythmias reported by the Great Ormond Street group could very well be due to damage to the sinus node by the suture line of the intra-atrial semisynthetic tunnel [6]. Furthermore, sick sinus syndrome, which may be caused by damage to the sinus node, carries a considerable risk of late sudden death. The course of the arterial supply of the sinus node in tricuspid atresia has been documented [9], but in other anomalies pertinent research has not been published to our knowledge.

DeLeval claims to have demonstrated that the contracting atrium only constitutes an extra resistance between the inferior caval vein to the crossroads of the right pulmonary artery and the superior caval vein. His experiments are very convincing, and analogous to known hydrodynamic principles that, surprisingly, were already put to practice in pre-Inca Peru [10]. The colleagues from the Mayo clinic maintain that the results with the 'classic' Fontan procedure are so good that they see no reason for change [11]. Furthermore, Puga and colleagues warn that the late desaturation of patients due to pulmonary arteriovenous fistula which has been described after partial [12–14] and total cavo-pulmonary connexions [15] may be due to the non-pulsatility of the pulmonary flow [16]. Nevertheless, the detailed and thorough analysis recently published by the Bordeaux and Birmingham groups is very disturbing, and constitutes a very good reason to scrutinize our long-term results [4]. Other problems with synthetic intracardiac tunnels in growing children are supportive of our aim to abolish the use of them whenever possible [17]. It is our opinion that the total cavo-pulmonary connexion with an intra-atrial tunnel constructed from the right auricle may well prove to be a good surgical option to reach that goal.

In conclusion we find that the use of the right auricle as an intercaval tunnel has two important advantages: firstly, no synthetic material is used, so that growth of the conduit is presumably no problem, just as in Senning procedures. Secondly, the sinus node and its blood supply are usually spared, so that perpetuation of sinus rhythm is to be expected.

Acknowledgement

We want to acknowledge H.J. Waterbolk for his artwork.

References

1. Puga FJ, Chiavarelli M, Hagler DJ (1987) Modifications of the Fontan operation applicable to patients with left atrioventricular valve atresia or single atrioventricular valve. Circulation 76 (suppl. III): 53–60.
2. DeLeval MR, Kilner P, Gewillig M, Bull C (1988) Total cavopulmonary connection for complex Fontan operations: experimental studies and early clinical experience. J Thorac Cardiovasc Surg 96: 682–695.
3. Jonas RA, Castaneda AR (1988) Modified Fontan procedure: atrial baffle and systemic venous to pulmonary artery anastomotic techniques. J Cardiac Surg 3: 91–96.

16

4. Fernandez G, Costa F, Fontan F, Naftel DC, Blackstone EH, Kirklin JW (1989) Prevalence of reoperation for pathway obstruction after Fontan operation. Ann Thorac Surg 48: 654–659.
5. Bink-Boelkens MTE, Bergstra A, Cromme-Dijkhuis AH, Eijgelaar A, Landsman MLJ, Mooyaart EL (1989) The asymptomatic child a long time after the Mustard operation for transposition of the great arteries. Ann Thorac Surg 47: 45–50.
6. Knott-Craig CJ (1989) Discussion of: Fontan F, Fernandez G, Costa F, et al. The size of the pulmonary arteries and the results of the Fontan operation. J Thorac Cardiovasc Surg 98: 719–720.
7. Humes RA, Feldt RH, Porter CJ, Julsrud PR, Puga FJ, Danielson GK (1988) The modified Fontan operation for asplenia and polysplenia syndromes. J Thorac Cardiovasc Surg 96: 212–218.
8. Matsuda H, Kawashima Y, Kishimoto H, et al. (1987) Problems in the modified Fontan operation for univentricular heart of the right ventricular type. Circulation 76 (suppl. III): 45–52.
9. Battistessa SA, Ho SY, Anderson RH, Smith A (1988) The arterial supply to the right atrium and the sinus node in classic tricuspid atresia. J Thorac Cardiovasc Surg 96: 816–822.
10. Ortloff CR (1988) Canal builders of pre-Inca Peru. Scientific American Dec 259: 74–80.
11. Puga FJ (1989) The modified Fontan operation [Letter to the editor]. J Thorac Cardiovasc Surg 98: 150.
12. Bargeron LM, Karp RB, Barcia A, Kirlin JW, Hunt DH, Deverall PB (1972) Late deterioration of patients after superior vena cava to right pulmonary artery anastomosis. Am J Cardiol 30: 211–216.
13. Mathur M, Glenn WWL (1973) Long-term evaluation of cavopulmonary artery anastomosis. Surgery 74: 899–916.
14. McFaul RC, Tajik AJ, Mair DD, Danielson GK, Seward JB (1977) Development of pulmonary arteriovenous shunt after superior vena cava-right pulmonary artery (Glenn) anastomosis: report of four cases. Circulation 55: 212–216.
15. Moore JW, Madden WA, Gaitner NS (1989) Development of pulmonary arteriovenous malformations after modified Fontan operations. J Thorac Cardiovasc Surg 98: 1045–1050.
16. Puga FJ (1989) Invited letter concerning: Pulmonary arteriovenous malformations after modified Fontan operation. J Thorac Cardiovasc Surg 98: 1144–1145.
17. Kirklin JW, Barrat-Boyes BG (1986) Cardiac Surgery. New York: John Wiley & Sons, 1183–1185.

The switch operation: indication and results

H. Meisner, S. Paek, R. Kunkel, W. Heimisch, Ch. Hähnel, H.P. Lorenz and
F. Sebening
The Heart Centre, Munich, F.R.G.

Looking back at the long history of surgical treatment of TGA it is obvious that there never was a problem of ingenuity, ideas or surgical know-how to treat such patients, but rather a problem of indication and understanding of hemodynamics together with development of surgical techniques and handling of such patients in the perioperative phase.

The good results with the atrial repair, e.g. Mustard or Senning, led to their general adoption up to the 1980s, when the arterial switch technique became more popular because of remarkably better results in the hands of a small number of surgeons. Controversy has continued as to whether the overall results of one operation are superior to those of the other. In that regard most of the early debate concerning the optimal treatment of infants with complete TGA centered on the surgical risks of the atrial switch as compared to the arterial switch procedures. We have to accept the fact that in the best hands the surgical mortality for the arterial procedure is still higher than that of an atrial inversion. As a matter of fact, the justification for anatomical correction is based on unsatisfactory long-term results of atrial inversion in patients with TGA. There is enough evidence that survival following an atrial repair of simple TGA after 20 yr will be between 70 and 88% [1-3], most patients being then in NYHA class 1. Two late complications, however, have raised concern as to the very long-term results of the Senning or Mustard repair. One is deteriorating right ventricular function, the other arrhythmia with sudden death.

The literature is filled with studies documenting right ventricular performance after such surgical procedures showing for instance an increased end-diastolic volume [4], or that both ejection fraction and response to exercise are decreased [5-7]. There are also reports [8], and we have seen it in some cases of our own experience, that right ventricular dysfunction may occur prior to surgery. Not only preoperative events but also perioperative management like improved neonatal resuscitation, earlier surgery or better myocardial preservation techniques may influence long-term outcome. There is some suggestion in the paper of Graham et al. [9] demonstrating a higher ejection fraction in patient groups operated on after 1975 compared to those before. Overall we have to accept a small number of late right heart failure, about 5% after 20 and more years, leaving for such patients as the only treatment cardiac transplantation or for a few the secondary switch operation according to Mee [10].

The considerable atrial surgery involved in the atrial inversion procedures appears to result in progressive loss of sinus rhythm. In our own experience of 306 patients with simple complete transposition undergoing Mustard's (n = 53) or more often Senning's (n = 253) operation over a period up to 16 yr 67% and 70% respectively are in sinus rhythm. The rest developed AV dissociation, AV block or paroxysmal and/or supraventricular tachycardia, in particular atrial flutter, which has a significant association with sudden death [11-13]. According to our experience sudden death is attributed to tachyarrhythmia rather than bradycardia, which cannot be solved by pacemaker treatment, at least not at the present stage of technical development. Generally one has to assume that 20 yr after an atrial inversion procedure more than 50% of the patients have lost their sinus rhythm, showing an intense inclination to development of atrial flutter [2,11,13]. There is a trend in our series towards better maintenance of sinus rhythm after the Senning procedure compared to the Mustard operation, but this difference is hampered by the divergent postoperative observation period (mean 8 yr versus 14 yr). Nevertheless sudden late death occurs in an unpredictable manner, since our ability to identify individuals at high risk is limited, at least at the current stage of electrophysiologic approach.

Overall and long-term experience with patients after the atrial switch support the continuous efforts to apply the arterial switch operation to all patients with TGA. There is general acceptance that the arterial switch operation represents better results for complex complete transposition, as it is evident from our own data (Fig. 1) that in these almost identical groups of patients the mortality is significantly lower in the switch series, even encountering the potential problem of comparing results obtained from patients operated upon several years before or more previously.

Although our early mortality with the Senning operation (see Fig. 2) in an

			mortality	
		n	early	late
1974 – 1983	Senning + correction	44	8(18.2%)	5(11.4%)
1983 – 7/1991	switch + correction	43	4(9.3%)	1(2.3%)

Fig. 1. Results of surgical treatment of patients with TGA and VSD, DORV and subpulmonary VSD and/or LVOTO (complex). The first group 1974-1983 was treated by atrial inversion, VSD closure etc., the second group with the switch operation.

identical age-group of newborns is much lower than with the switch procedure, we are favoring this approach for simple transposition as it is done in an increasing number of centers. Without doubt the arterial switch procedure is a more demanding and difficult surgical procedure; the achieved results depend according to our opinion on the experience of the team, that is anesthetist, cardiac surgeon and intensivist; certainly an exact diagnosis should be provided by an experienced cardiologist.

Today we see the indication for a switch operation in simple TGA in the first weeks of life and all cases with TGA and VSD and special forms of DORV and subpulmonary VSD and LVOTO. We do see contraindications in the case of a tunnel-type LVOTO or if the aortic valve shows malformations – not bicuspidal-isation –, if A-V valve anomalies are present or special forms of coronary pattern like type AB 2 or intramural course make the transfer more hazardous (Table 1).

We prefer to repair simple complete TGA anatomically in the first 2 wk of life and not later than 1 mth of age; the left ventricle will manage a systemic work load; in our series age at operation varied between 2 and 36 days, mean 11 days. In the complex group age varied between 8 and 4933 days, mean 156 days. All patients with simple TGA were kept on prostaglandin E_1, with the intention to

Table 1. Listing of indications and contraindications to the arterial switch operations in patients with TGA

Indication	Contraindication
Simple TGA + PDA < 6 wk old	LVOTO (tunnel)
TGA + VSD	Aortic valve stenosis
TGA + LVOTO (functional)	A-V valve disease
DORV (Taussig - Bing)	Coronary pattern (intramural)
DORV, sup. - inf. V., VSD	
TrA - IIc (TGA)	

		n	mortality
1979 – 7/1991	Senning	44	–
1985 – 7/1991	switch	73	3(4.1%)

Fig. 2. Results of surgical therapy of comparable groups of newborns with simple TGA operated on either by atrial or arterial inversion.

rehypertrophy the perhaps already involuted left ventricle. From cardiac catheterisation pressure data were available; in our series at this time the ratio was on average 0.84 (Table 2).

2-D echocardiography showed the left ventricular posterior wall thickness to be on average systolic 6 mm and diastolic 4 mm at least. Septum geometry was analysed according to shape; left ventricular mass was correlated to left ventricular enddiastolic volume, the ratio being normal between 1.3 and 1.7 [14]. The Doppler flow signal across the mitral valve (> 1 m/s) corresponds to an open duct and should be larger than the tricuspid flow.

If a patient does not fulfill these criteria or the infant is referred to our center after the neonatal period or multiorgan failure persists, and prematurity or late development of right ventricular dysfunction contraindicates correction at the atrial level, preparations for a two-stage arterial procedure will be discussed.

Table 2. Summary of preoperative data and functional measurements mandatory for decision-making in newborns with simple TGA

Age	< 6 wk
$P \dfrac{LV}{RV}$	< 0.6
LV wall thickness	syst. 6 mm diast. 4 mm
Septum geometry	shape index 1:1
$LV \dfrac{mass}{volume}$	1.3-1.7
Flow mitral	1 m/s

Results

All patients with TGA admitted to our hospital were submitted to cardiac catheterisation (Klinik f. Herz – und Kreislauferkrankungen im Kindesalter, Dir. Prof. Dr. K. Bühlmeyer). During that procedure a Rashkind manoeuvre was performed. The effect on oxygen saturation is depicted in Fig. 3.

In TGA and VSD there is an average increase of 14%, in DORV 9% and in simple TGA 18.1%

Since our first arterial switch procedure for a patient with DORV (Taussig Bing) in May 12, 1983, at age 11 mth (prior banding, coarctation resection and ASE at 4 days and 5 months) till July 1991, 117 patients have been operated on; 71% were male, 29% female. Preoperatively 21% of the infants with simple TGA were intubated and ventilated, 89% received prostaglandin E_1, 67% had diuretics. Weight at operation in the group with simple TGA was 2.2-4.2 kg (mean 3.3 kg), for the complex cases 4-56 kg (mean 14.2 kg). Overall mortality was 6.8%

(cf. Fig. 4). The causes of death are listed in Table 3; myocardial death due to ischemia and invisible coronary problems were predominant. Two patients died late of noncardiac causes. Age at operation and early mortality of newborns and simple TGA is depicted in fig. 5; no correlation, however, could be demonstrated.

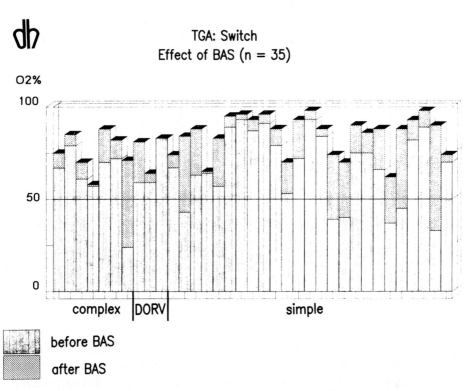

Fig. 3. Actual data of O$_2$ % increase after the Rashkind procedure of 35 consecutive patients with TGA. The first 7 patients had complex forms of TGA, 3 had DORV-Taussig Bing malformation and 25 were simple TGA. The effects of BAS were quite variable.

Table 3. Causes of hospital and late death after the switch operation (*n* = 117) between May 1983 and July 1991

Diagnosis	*n*	Time	Causes
TGA	2	op	Intramural
TGA + CoA	1	op	Myocardial
TGA + VSD	2	op	Myocardial
Taussig–Bing	1	1 day	Myocardial
TGA, VSD + CoA (no op)	1	14 days	Renal
2-stage-op TGA	1	24 days	Cardiac insuff.
TGA, VSD (Debanding)	1	226 days	Pulm. hypert.
TGA	1	370 days	CNS

diagnosis	n	early	$\mp$ %	late
intact VS	73	3	4.1	1
2−stage−op	1	1	−	−
+ VSD	23	3	⎫ 10.3	1
complex	6	−	⎬	−
T.−Bing	14	1	7.1	−
	117	8	6.8	2

Fig. 4. Results after the arterial switch operation in the Heart Center, Munich, between March 1983 and July 31, 1991.

Mean cardiopulmonary bypass time was 147 min (84–387 min) in simple TGA and 183 min (119–399 min) in the complex cases; the mean period of aortic cross-clamping was 99 min (66–177 min) and 127 min (80–180) respectively. The duration of cardiopulmonary bypass was not identified as a risk factor because long times were generally the results of problems rather than the cause.

Surgical technique

The technique of the arterial switch operation is based on the experience of Quaegebeur et al. [15] with small variations evolved during the past years [16]. We use continuous extracorporal perfusion at flows of 2.5 l/min/m^2, the patient is cooled to 17–19°C, reducing flow at that temperature by half. Cold Bretschneider solution is infused as cardioplegia (5–10 ml/g heart weight). The coronary arteries are transferred using a button or a scallop of the aortic wall containing the coronary ostium. Since the beginning we have used absorbable suture material (PDS) and never have observed any problems. The defects in the neopulmonary artery are filled by suturing into place pieces of autologous pericardium that have been recently prepared for 10 min in glutaraldehyde, which makes it easier to manipulate. In cases where the sinus of Valsava are destroyed by the excision of the coronary arteries we use a large 'pantaloon' patch of pericardium for reconstruction [17]. In all patients, the Lecompte manoeuvre was applied, even in side-by-side position of the great arteries (except one). We never had to insert a conduit. Generally there are no technical difficulties in performing the switch operation.

When a VSD is present, it is usually repaired before the actual switch operation is begun. In 45% the VSD was closed by the transatrial approach, in 30% through the pulmonary artery or the aorta, occasionally a repair through the right ventricle was indicated; 8% of the group with simple TGA had an insignificant VSD, which was closed by one stitch only.

During the rewarming and weaning off bypass phase anesthesia management becomes a significant part. The sudden changes of load conditions to the left ventricle after the switch operation present a hazardous event. In our hands (Dr. Kunkel) the application of phentolamine, a short-acting alpha-blocker, in repetitive doses of 1 mg (up to 4–5 mg) during the rewarming phase yielding perfusion pressures below 50 mmHg, provided optimal load conditions for the immediate postbypass phase. Circulatory support is mandatory in almost all patients in the early peri- and postoperative period using dobutamine up to 10 µg/kg/min and dopamine 3 µg/kg/min. The high dose of dobutamine is necessary

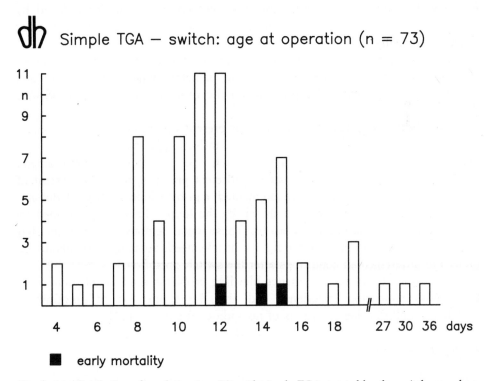

Fig. 5. Age distribution of newborns (*n* = 73) with simple TGA, treated by the switch procedure, and early mortality.

only in the first 30 min after cardiopulmonary bypass; generally it can be reduced to 5 µg/kg/min, a dose which we continue for the next few days on the intensive care unit. Dopamine (3 µg/kg/min) is always administered from the beginning of operation throughout the procedure, thus avoiding renal problems.

A more comprehensive evaluation and assessment of the hemodynamic response to the different physiological state in this critical phase was achieved by intraoperative registration of ventricular function using sonomicrometry [18]. Piezoelectric crystals were mounted on a small dacron patch and attached to the anterior and posterior epicardial surface of both ventricles with fibrin glue. Repetitive transit time measurements (1000 times per second) of ultrasound travelling along an anterior – posterior axis registered the diameter changes and thus the contraction pattern of each ventricle simultaneously and continuously. Pressure in each ventricular cavity was recorded by a needle-tipped manometer for cyclic correlation. The original curves recorded in a 3730 g newborn are depicted in Fig. 6. Left ventricular (RV) (Fig. 6a) and right ventricular pressures (LV) (Fig. 6b) and the diameter of the corresponding chamber are compared with the same parameters after the switch operation. Before surgical correction the LVP was 40/5 mmHg, immediately after the switch procedure, during steady-state conditions at the end of extracorporeal circulation, the pressure in the LV was systemic (70/5 mmHg) and in the RV 40/5 mmHg. Ventricular function, however, has not yet recovered, showing contraction amplitudes reduced by almost 40%. Increasing preload and infusion of dobutamine improved ventricular function markedly.

In the lower part of the figures the cyclic pressure diameter relations are shown as an *x-y* plot, generating the loops from the diameter signal on the abscissa and the corresponding ventricular pressure on the ordinate in a counterclockwise direction.

Beat-to-beat recordings of these variables present a pressure-diameter diagram, the area of such (pressure times distance) reflecting in part the stroke work produced by the ventricles. After the switch operation, the pressure-diameter loops of the left ventricle demonstrate sufficient pressure, but a low extent of systolic shortening, which can be augmented, e.g. by administration of dobutamine and increase of preload. As shown by the loops, the work performed by each ventricle is markedly increased. These data demonstrate that the left ventricle in particular, but also the right ventricle, needs some time for adaptation under the different load conditions after the switch operation.

In the beginning of our experience bleeding problems used to consume some time. With increasing experience and also the application of aprotinin, a proteinase inhibitor, hemostasis is of no additional concern [19].

Postoperative care

All patients were ventilated after operation in the ICU; for simple TGA 2-28 days, mean 6.2 days; for the complex group 0-60 days, mean 9.8. Catecholamine

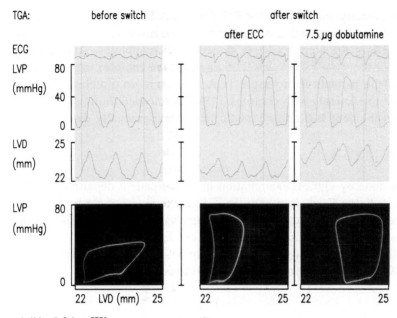

pat.: H.A. ♂, 8 days, 3730 g

Fig. 6. (a) Original tracings of LV pressure and diameter changes in a newborn before and after the switch operation using sonomicrometry. The lower part of the figure shows an *x-y* plot of diameter and pressure signal reflecting stroke work.

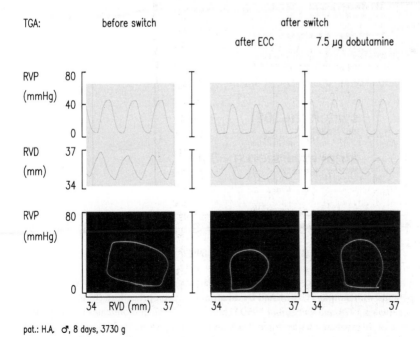

pat.: H.A. ♂, 8 days, 3730 g

Fig. 6. (b) Original curves of the right ventricle in the same infant (see text).

26

support was neccessary on average for 6.5 days. In 11% of the newborns the application of nitrates was indicated because of persisting elevated left atrial pressure: only 3% of the complex cases showed such symptoms. Average stay in the hospital for the simple TGA was 21.5 days, for the complex cases 31 days. At discharge of the patients with simple TGA 27% were on diuretics and 22% had digitalis. Of the patients with complex TGA 50% needed diuretics and 58% digitalis. Within the next 1-6 mth all medications were gradually discontinued.

Late results

Follow-up was done by clinical examination in the outpatient department of the Department of Pediatric Cardiology (Dir. Prof. K. Bühlmeyer) of our hospital and correspondence and telephone calls with referring physicians and families of the patients. All patients operated on before December 31, 1990, were traced and the last date of follow-up was between June and July 31, 1991. The median time of follow up is 39.5 mth, with a range from 7 to 91 mth.

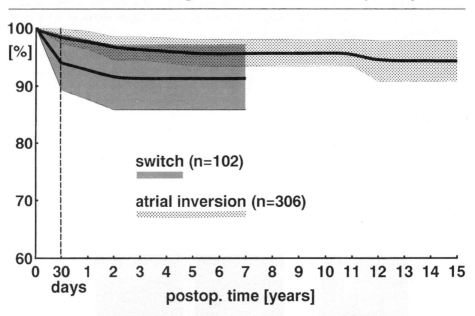

Fig. 7. Actuarial survival calculated to the method of Kaplan and Meier. The first curve concerns the data of 306 patients with simple TGA treated by an atrial inversion procedure (Mustard *n* = 53, Senning *n* = 253) between 1974 and December 1990. The second curve demonstrates survival after the switch operation of 63 neonates with simple TGA and 39 complex cases between May 1983 and December 1990. The shaded areas represent the 70% confidence limits of the actuarial estimates.

Late survival

The 32-mth actuarial survival rate including both early and late deaths was 89.4%. There were 2 late deaths, after 226 and 370 days respectively; the one due to progressive pulmonary hypertension after banding and then VSD closure and the other to cerebral seizures due to late postoperative sepsis (cf. Fig. 7).

Post-repair left ventricular function, assessed by two-dimensional echocardiography, was impaired in about 5% in the first days after operation, normalizing postoperatively within weeks to months. 92% had normal left ventricular dimensions in a late postoperative study [14], except one patient with pulmonary hypertension who had in addition an occluded right coronary artery.

Minor gradients from the right ventricle to the pulmonary artery were measured in more than half the cases using two-dimensional and Doppler echocardiography. There is no doubt that this method overestimates in these patients the actual gradients because of an unfavourable measuring angle and eddy formation in the dilatated pulmonary artery bifurcation. Either no or only a small (< 20 mmHg) gradient was present in 44 patients (73%), 5 had a gradient between 21 and 40 mmHg and only 2 (3.3%) showed a gradient of 41 and 60 mmHg in the group of simple TGA.

Among the 95 surviving patients 3 have clinical and ultrasonic evidence of neoaortic valvular incompetence; one is mild and two are very small. Two patients gave evidence of neopulmonary valvular insufficiency of minor degree.

Sinus rhythm was present in 100% of the patients with simple TGA and 89% after complex TGA repair; in the latter group 4 needed a pacemaker.

None of the patients after simple TGA correction has required reoperation up to now. Among the complex cases one patient (2.8%) underwent repair of a residual VSD; five other patients are under observation because of insignificant residual VSDs.

Of all the 95 surviving patients 92 were in NYHA Class 1 at the time of the last follow-up and three in NYHA Class 2. Only two patients of the complex group and one with simple TGA are on digitalis and/or diuretics; that is 95% without any medication showing normal physical and mental development.

Discussion

Certainly surgical treatment offers the only effective therapy to patients with TGA, because only 15% of all newborns with simple TGA survive the first 6 months of life. The history of surgery for TGA started in 1950 [16], leaving today after 40 years of intense development two possible modes of surgical treatment for this anomaly: on the one hand physiologic repair by intraatrial rerouting of venous return providing a dramatic increase of life expectancy, albeit late right ventricular dysfunction, dysrhythmias, and concern about the function of the tricuspid valve cause apprehension about their functional capacity. On the other hand a more demanding and difficult procedure, the arterial switch operation, has proven to offer better results in cases with complex TGA [41], whereas in simple TGA satisfactory results can only be achieved by operating in the newborn period but with a higher operative mortality [38–40]. Thus the hazard of death is highest for the switch procedure at the time of operation; for the atrial switch the risk of late deaths due to arrhythmia is predominant in our series after 2, 4 and 11 years (Fig. 8).

Concerning the imperfection of the atrial inversion procedures (Mustard or Senning) the literature is filled with detailed information regarding late functional results. We have to accept the following facts:

1. After 10 and more years arrhythmia presents a risk of death in about 10% of the patients [1,2,13,29].

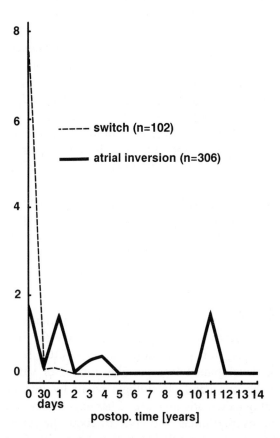

Hazard of death after surgical correction of TGA (n=408)

----- switch (n=102)

▬ atrial inversion (n=306)

postop. time [years]

Fig. 8. Hazard function of the same patient cohort; time zero is the time of entrance of the patient into the pediatric cardiac center. The hazard of death is highest for the switch operation at the time of operation; for the atrial inversion procedures there are a number of late deaths.

2. Objective evaluation of RV function reveals an abnormal response to exercise in some patients. There are reports of terminal right heart failure in a few patients 15-20 or more years after atrial switch [3,7,20,28].

3. There is no doubt that the morphological and muscular structures of the left and right ventricle are different. We do have a variety of reasons to assume that the muscular function of the RV will never last as long as the LV, e.g. the stratum compactum to stratum spongiosum ratio is 3:1 in the LV and 1:3 in the RV and the compact layer is more responsible for contraction rather than the trabecular spongiosum layer. The left ventricle has two well-developed coronary arteries. The papillary muscles are very different; thus the tensor apparatus of the LV is much better suited to perform systemic hemodynamic work than is the tensor apparatus of the right ventricle [21]. To this effect congenital corrected transposition (CCTGA) offers an experimental model set up by nature, though in rare instances without associated cardiac anomalies. These individuals do reasonably well during the first few decades of life, developing then in 30% severe and lethal arrhythmias [22]. Although an actual estimate of survival is difficult, there is an increasing rate of death from chronic congestive heart failure beginning in the third and fifth decades of life [24]. There are reports [23,37] that on exercise in this group of patients the ejection fraction of the LV increases, but not in the RV, being still better than in patients after atrial inversion.

Overall experience with patients after atrial switch and these more theoretical thoughts support the continuous efforts to apply the arterial switch operation for correction of patients with transposition of the great arteries. The indication is given in TGA and VSD or DORV and subpulmonary VSD, or cases with membranous or functional LVOTO. These anomalies of variable morphology usually complicate management of TGA presenting also a variety of additional cardiac anomalies. According to reports from other centers [3,15,25,26] and our own experience (cf. Fig. 1), there is a lower mortality and morbidity as compared to atrial switch because the left ventricle is trained to sustain the systemic workload without particular problems. For this group we favour primary correction within the first 3-4 months of life, provided no coarctation or interrupted aortic arch needs repair in advance. Meanwhile, a low operative risk and satisfactory short-term survival are reported from experienced centers in that group of patients [27]. Even though Björk and Bouchart [16] realized, as well as Mustard in 1954, that a high left ventricular pressure is required for a successful 'switchover' anastomosis, it took more than 20 years for this procedure to be generally accepted as treatment for infants with intact ventricular septum. Today the usual patient with isolated TGA is considered a candidate for arterial repair in the first 4-6 weeks of life. In our hospital we prefer the administration of PGE, in order to increase volume and work load of the left ventricle. We also still prefer angiography, mostly connected with BAS, for exclusion of additional malformations, demonstration of morphology and coronary anatomy. Based on such data the operative strategy can be arranged and handling of the parents becomes easier. According to Kirklin et al. in the congenital Heart Surgeons

Society-TGA study, operative risk increases with age, being higher in the third and later weeks of life. Our experience (Fig. 5) could not support these findings, but as shown we prefer operative correction within the first 2 weeks of life. The operative technique has been standardized meanwhile. Extensive dissection of the pulmonary vessels avoided implantation of conduits or foreign material. Coronary ostia transfer can be accomplished in a standardized fashion. Intramural course, which is in our opinion a contraindication to the switch procedure, can mostly be recognized only after dissection of the aorta. In our experience coronary pattern type AB 2 is connected with a higher mortality (3 of 5 died), depending on the position and rotation of the great vessels to each other, e.g. when the pulmonary artery is more posterior there is a higher risk. The possibility of using an internal mammary artery bypass for perfusion [30,31] is recognized, but has to be regarded as a 'bail-out' procedure rather than a common surgical technique. In our experience anesthesia and intraoperative handling deserve a great deal of consideration providing at the end of extracorporeal circulation a low peripheral resistance to the left ventricle. In almost all cases of simple TGA and switch operation catecholamine support of variable dose, e.g. dopamine (3 µg/kg/min) and dobutamine (5–10 µg/kg/min), is mandatory. As we have shown by intra-operative measurements (Fig. 6), the ventricle needs some time and support for adaptation.

The late results in the literature emphasize a high rate of RV–PA gradients, but of minor degree. Very probably they are caused by undue tension of the pulmonary branches or subpulmonary muscular stenosis. According to Paillole et al. this can be improved by liberal implantation of a large pericardial patch. Valve incompetence especially of the neoaorta is rare, perhaps caused by dilatation of the aortic ring in connection with coronary ostia implantation. Depending on the technique used, Yamaguchi et al. [32] for instance describe a higher rate of aortic incompetence (28%) if U-shaped defects were created instead of button-holes (8%) for coronary reimplantation. For a certain group of patients the two-stage operation can be considered, whereas for some a training period for the left ventricle by banding of several months has been required [33,34], lately. Jonas et al. [35] published promising results after a short training interval of about 9 days only.

Still the overall mortality of this operation is about 10% [25,36]. According to the literature [15,25,39,40] and our own experience, the causes of late death are myocardial ischemia and in a few instances progressive pulmonary hypertension. At the moment there is no doubt that we have to accept a higher surgical mortality for the arterial switch operation in simple TGA. The long-term results are promising but do not exceed a decade of experience. According to our experience optimal therapy is based on a precise and selfcritical pre- and intraoperative management combined with excellent intensive-care conditions.

Summary

In view of the reports on late complications after atrial rerouting and improved early mortality after the arterial switch operation the latter gains significance in treating patients with TGA. Beginning in May 1983, 117 patients with an overall mortality of 6.8% have been operated on. Two children died late due to non-cardiac complications. In the late follow-up small gradients in the RV outflow tract have been measured by Doppler echocardiography; in a few patients semilunar valvar incompetence has been recognized. Up to now none of the patients with simple TGA required reoperation.

Currently we see an indication for the switch operation in TGA and VSD and related forms of complex malformations, but also in simple TGA within the newborn period. Contraindications are the LVOTO-tunnel stenoses, severe valve malformations or special types of the coronary artery pattern.

References

1. Williams WG, Trusler GA, Kirklin JW, Blackstone EH, Coles JG, Izukawa T (1988) Early and late results of a protocol for simple transposition leading to an atrial switch (Mustard) repair. J Thorac Cardiovasc Surg 95: 717-726.
2. Turina M, Siebenmann R, Nussbaumer P, Senning A (1988) Longterm outlook after atrial correction for transposition of great arteries: cautious optimism. J Thorac Cardiovasc Surg 95: 828-835.
3. Turina M, von Segesser L, Schönbeck M, Bauer E, Laske A, Senning A (1991) Atriale Korrektur der Transposition der grossen Arterien (TGA): Langzeitergebnisse und Spätproblematik. J Thorac Cardiovasc Surg 39: 57.
4. Hagler DJ, Ritter DG, Mair DD, Tajik AJ, Seward JB, Fulton RE, Ritmann EL (1979) Right and left ventricular function after the Mustard procedure for transposition of the great arteries. Am J Cardiol 44: 276-283.
5. Hurwitz RA, Caldwell RL, Girod DA, Mahony L, Brawn J, King H (1985) Ventricular function in transposition of the great arteries: evaluation by radionuclide angiocardiographie. Am Heart J 110: 600-605.
6. Shimazaki Y, Kawashima Y, Ogawa M, Hirose H, Miyamoto K, Morimoto S (1985) Right and left ventricular volume characteristics in children with transposition of the great arteries after Mustard's procedure. Jpn Circ J 49: 679-684.
7. Ramsay JM, Venables AW, Kelly MJ, Kalff V (1984) Right and left ventricular function at rest and with exercise after the Mustard operation for transposition of the great arteries. Br Heart J 51: 364-370.
8. Jaymakani JMM, Canent RV (1974) Preoperative and postoperative right ventricular function in children with transposition of the great arteries. Circulation 50: 1139-1145.
9. Graham TP, Burger J, Bender HW, Hammon JW, Boucek RJ, Appleton S (1985) Improved right ventricular function after intra-atrial repair of transposition of the great arteries. Circulation 72: 1145-1151.
10. Mee RBB (1986) Severe right ventricular failure after Mustard or Senning operation. J Thorac Cardiovasc Surg 92: 385-390.
11. Deanfield JE, Cullen S, Gewillig M (1991) Arrhythmias after surgery for complete transposition: do they matter? Cardiol Young 1: 91-96.

32

12. Deanfield JE, Camm J, Macartney F, Cartwright T, Douglas J, Drew J, de Leval M, Stark J (1988) Arrhythmia and late mortality after Mustard and Senning operation for transposition of the great arteries: an eight year prospective study. J Thorac Cardiovasc Surg 96: 569-576.
13. Hayes CJ, Gersony WM (1986) Arrhythmias after the Mustard operation for TGA: a longterm study. J Am Coll Cardiol 7: 133-137.
14. Vogel M, Meisner H, Smallhorn JF, Bühlmeyer K (1991) The role of myocardial perfusion scintigraphy and echocardiographic wall motion analysis in the postoperative assessment of patients after the arterial switch operation. In: TGA 25 years after Rashkind Balloon Septostomy; Symposium Munich, May 3-5, Springer-Breitkopf Verlag.
15. Quaegebeur JM, Rohmer J, Ottenkamp J, Buis T, Kirklin JW, Blackstone EH, Brom AG (1986) The arterial switch operation. J Thorac Cardiovasc Surg 92: 361-384.
16. Meisner H, Sebening F (1991) Transposition der grossen Arterien, einschliesslich korrigierte Transposition. Kirschnersche allgemeine u. spezielle Operationslehre, Band VI/2, Herzchirurgie. Berlin-Heidelberg: Springer-Verlag.
17. Paillole C, Sidi D, Kachaner J, Planché C, Belot JP, Villain E, Le Bidois J, Piéchaud JF, Pedroni E (1988) Fate of pulmonary artery after anatomic correction of simple transposition of great arteries in newborn infants. Circulation 78: 870-876.
18. Heimisch W (1987) Dynamic changes in regional geometry and coherent myocardial contraction vectors of the left ventricle assessed by sonomicrometry. In: HP Kimmich and MR Neuman, eds. Biotelemetry IX, Braunschweig: Döring-Druck, 117-120.
19. Mössinger H, Dietrich W, Spannagel M, Jochum M, Richter JA (1991) Influence of Aprotinin on coagulation patterns and blood loss in infants undergoing surgery for congenital heart defects. Anesthesiology Suppl, Sept.
20. Redington AN (1991) Functional assessment of the heart after corrective surgery for complete transposition. Cardiol Young 1: 84-90.
21. van Praagh R (1991) The arterial switch operation in d-transposition of the great arteries: anatomic indications and contraindications. J Thorac Cardiovasc Surg 39: 53.
22. Huhta JC, Maloney JD, Ritter DG, Ilstrup DM, Feldt RH (1983) Complete atrioventricular block in patients with atrioventricular discordance. Circulation 67: 1374.
23. Peterson R, Franck RH, Fajmann WA, Jones RH (1988) Comparison of cardiac function in surgically corrected and congenitally corrected transposition of the great arteries. J Thorac Cardiovasc Surg 96: 227-236.
24. Graham TP, Parrish MD, Boucek RJ, Boerth RC, Breitweser JA, Thompson S, Robertson RM, Morgan JR, Griesinger GC (1983) Assessment of ventricular size and function in congenitally corrected transposition of the great arteries. Am J Cardiol 51: 245.
25. Castaneda AR, Trusler GA, Paul MH, Blackstone EH, Kirklin JW (1988) The early results of treatment of simple transposition in the current era. J Thorac Cardiovasc Surg 95: 14-28.
26. Kirklin JW (1991) The surgical repair for complete transposition. Cardiol Young 1: 13-25.
27. Comas JV, Serraf A, Lacour-Gayet F, Bruniaux J, Bouchart F, Planché C (1991) Neonatal anatomic repair of TGA and VSD. EACTS 5th annual meeting, London, Sept, Abstract 29.
28. Colan SD, Trowitzsch E, Wernovsky G, Sholler GF, Sanders SP, Castaneda AR (1988) Myocardial performance after arterial switch operation for transposition of the great arteries with intact ventricular septum. Circulation 78: 132-141.
29. Flinn CJ, Wolff GS, Dick M (1984) Cardiac rhythm after the Mustard operation for complete transposition of the great arteries. N Engl J Med 310: 1635-1638.
30. Ebels T, Meuzelaar K, Gallandat Huet RCG, Bink-Boelkens MTE, Cromme-Dijkhuis A, Bams JL, Boeve WJ, Eijgelaar A (1989) Neonatal arterial switch operation complicated by intramural left coronary artery and treated by left internal mammary artery bypass graft. J Thorac Cardiovasc Surg 97: 473-475.
31. Rheuban KS, Kron IL, Bulatovic A (1990) Internal mammary artery bypass after the arterial switch operation. Ann Thorac Surg 50: 125-126.

32. Yamaguchi M, Hosokawa Y, Imai Y, Kurosawa H, Yasui H, Yagihara T, Okamoto F, Wakaki N (1990) Early and midterm results of the arterial switch operation for transposition of the great arteries in Japan. J Thorac Cardiovasc Surg 100: 261-269.

33. Lange PE, Pulss W, Sievers HH, Wessel A, Onnasch DGW, Bernhard A, Yacoub MH, Heintzen PH (1986) Cardiac rhythm and conduction after two-stage anatomic correction of simple transposition of the great arteries. Thorac Cardiovasc Surg 34: 22-24.

34. Lange PE, Sievers HH, Onnasch DGW, Yacoub MH, Bernhard A, Heintzen PH (1986) Up to 7 years of follow-up after two-stage anatomic correction of simple transposition of the great arteries. Circulation 74: Suppl I, 1-47.

35. Jonas RA (1991) Update on the rapid two-stage arterial switch procedure. Cardiol Young 1: 99.

36. Nakazawa M, Oyama K, Imai Y, Nojima K, Aotsuka H, Satomi G, Kurosawa H, Takao A (1988) Criteria for two-staged arterial switch operation for simple transposition of great arteries. Circulation 78: 124-131.

37. Mathews RA, Fricker FJ, Beermann LB, Stephenson RJ, Fischer DR, Neches WH, Park SC, Lenox CC, Zuberbuhler JR (1983) Exercise studies after the Mustard operation in transposition of the great arteries. Am J Cardiol 51: 1526-1536.

38. Wernovsky G, Hougen TJ, Walsh EP, Sholler GF, Colan SD, Sanders SP, Parness IA, Keane JF, Mayer JE, Jonas RA, Castaneda AR, Lang P (1988) Midterm results after the arterial switch operation for transposition of the great arteries with intact ventricular septum: clinical, hemodynamic, echocardiographic, and electrophysiologic data. Circulation 77: 1333-1344.

39. Mee RBB (1991) Results of the arterial switch procedure for complete transposition with an intact ventricular septum. Cardiol Young 1: 97.

40. Norwood WI, Dobell AR, Freed MD, Kirklin JW, Blackstone EH (1988) Intermediate results of the arterial switch repair. J Thorac Cardiovasc Surg 96: 854-863.

41. Sidi D, Planché C, Kachaner J, Bruniaux J, Villain E, le Bidois J, Piéchaud J-F, Lacour-Gayet F (1987) Anatomic correction of simple transposition of the great arteries in 50 neonates. Circulation 75: 429-435.

Significance of myocardial predamage and condition in ischemic tolerance of the heart

H.J. Bretschneider and M.M. Gebhard

Zentrum Physiologie and Pathophysiologie, Göttingen University, F.R.G.

The significance of preischemic conditions for the tolerance of the heart to ischemia can, in our opinion, only be properly understood if the course of a complete global cardiac ischemia is analysed as follows: (1) according to the three main reversible phases; (2) according to the time-related development of damage and subsequent recovery; and (3) according to the three crucial pathophysiological processes involved.

Figure 1a shows the three phases of a reversible ischemia. For our purposes, it is of importance to note that up to the end of the first phase, reperfusion immediately results in full function; in the second phase, during which the phosphocreatine breaks down, the time of recovery increases linearly; and during the third phase an increasingly steep rise in the recovery time takes place, becoming almost exponential [2–4].

Figure 1b, taken from a recent publication by Gebhard, shows the dependence of recovery time on the degree of damage, which is of vital importance [9]. The degree of damage in the course of global ischemia shows a sigmoid increase. At first, there is no significant injury but then the curve bends sharply upwards, finally levelling off when damage asymptotically approaches the irreversible state. The dotted lines and the corresponding arrows parallel to the abscissa indicate the exponential rise in recovery time over the steep part of the curve for ischemic damage.

This picture gives rise to two questions. First: Can the curve be shifted to the right by favourable measures or to the left by unfavourable conditions? The answer is yes, in actual fact to a great extent! A shift to the right is brought about by, among other things, a diminished energy requirement before arrest of the heart, a low temperature during ischemia and a favourable cardioplegia and myocardial protection. Conversely, a higher energy requirement before cardiac arrest, a high temperature during ischemia and a less favourable myocardial protection would produce a shift to the left.

The second question is: Why does the damage not develop linearly with duration of ischemia? Can this typical sigmoid course of ischemia-dependent damage during heart surgery be made linear, perhaps by use of pharmacological or biochemical tricks? The answer to this is that the sigmoid course, being a fundamental natural phenomenon, cannot be changed – it can only be shifted to the left or to the right. It is true that certain parameters of cell damage, for instance, cellular swelling, follow a fairly linear path. However, as a result of the

36

interaction between several crucial ischemia-dependent processes, the characteristic sigmoid shape is always found, along with a recovery time corresponding to the degree of damage. The three crucial pathophysiological processes taking place during ischemia are: development of acidosis, due to anaerobiosis; swelling of cells and organelles, due to overtaxing of the osmotic regulation; and the progressive decrease in energy status.

These three processes are complementary to each other, also in their effect on an increasing structural damage, as shown in the schema in Fig. 2a [10]. Figure 2b demonstrates that development of acidosis in the extracellular space does not

Definition by functional criteria	Biochemical equivalent	Latency period of recovery and period of recovery
I. Period of latency	Consumption of the O_2-pool; no production of lactate	no latency of recovery, no recovery time
II. Period of increasing disturbances in function up to complete paralysis	Breakdown of PKr; small decrease of ATP; production of lactate	no significant patency of recovery; increase of recovery time proportional to the decreasing PKr-content
III. Duration of the total but still-reversible loss of functions	Breakdown of ATP to 60% of the normal initial value; further production of lactate	latency of recovery, exponential increase of the recovery time proportional to the decreasing ATP-content

Fig. 1. (a) The three periods of the reanimation time of the heart. From Bretschneider et al., 1975 [4].

ISCHEMIC DAMAGE [%]

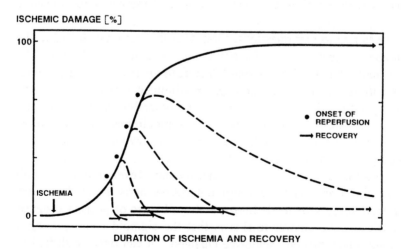

DURATION OF ISCHEMIA AND RECOVERY

Fig. 1. (b) The relationship between duration of ischemia, duration of recovery from ischemia, and ischemia damage. From Gebhard, 1990 [9].

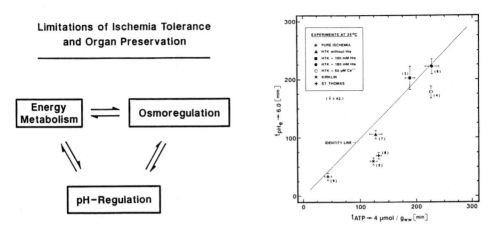

Fig. 2. (a) From Gebhard, 1992 [10]. (b) From Gebhard, 1987 [7].

always correspond to a decrease in energy status. Here, the time taken to reach an ATP concentration of 4 $\mu M/g_{ww}$ and the time taken to reach a pH value of 6.0 in the dog myocardium at 25°C under varying conditions of cardioplegia are plotted against each other [7]. The values for pure ischemia or our method of myocardial protection lie on the identity line, whereas addition of calcium ions to our solution and other methods of cardioplegia cause greater acidosis in relation to the maintenance of energy status. A relatively high degree of acidosis is, in our experience, often accompanied by severe intracellular oedema.

The dependence of cellular oedema on the degree of acidosis is also observed in the capillary endothelium, as shown by morphometric studies on the heart.

During pure ischemia, and during ischemia under protection according to Kirklin, with the solution developed by St. Thomas' Hospital and with HTK solution, an increase in the average thickness of the endothelium to almost double its value takes place, when the pH drops below 6.0 at 25°C. This is largely independent of the method of protection, although the time taken for development of acidosis to pH 6.0 varies by up to a factor of 7, as seen in Fig. 3b. The swelling of the endothelium and of the myocytes as well as of their organelles, particularly the mitochondria, is evidence for the overtaxing of the osmotic or volume regulation under ischemic conditions [5].

Figure 4a shows the changes in the surface-to-volume ratios of the mitochondria for pure ischemia and for ischemia protected by St. Thomas' solution and by HTK solution [11]. The time course is very similar and fairly constant under all three sets of conditions. With regard to the absolute niveau, however, there are considerable differences which can be traced back to differences in outward transport of lactic acid, in exchange between sodium and hygrogen ions and in the supply of anaerobic energy. Intracellular oedema (in Fig. 4b) characterized by the free sarcoplasm of the myocytes increases parallel to the decrease in the surface-volume relationship of the mitochondria. The myocyte swelling reaches

38

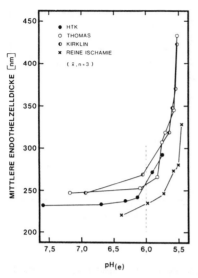

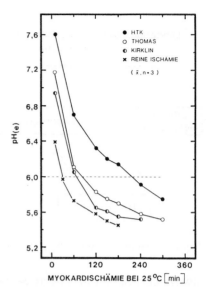

Fig. 3. (a) Dependence of the average endothelium-cell capillary thickness on the interstitial pH-value in the myocardium of the dog at a global ischemia at 25°C. It has been protectively pretreated either with the Kirklin-solution, the St-Thomas-Hospital-solution, or with the HTK-solution. The discontinued line marks the pH-value of 6.0, the value critical for myocardial resuscitation. (b) Development of acidosis at 25°C in ischemic dog-myocardium while implementing various protective measures; the cardioplegic method according to Kirklin, St-Thomas-Hospital, and Bretschneider. The discontinued line specifies the pH-value of 6.0, critical for myocardial resuscitation.

its final value first, however. Particularly impressive is the rapid development of cellular oedema for pure ischemia [11].

Now, by what factors or avoidable mistakes in the pre-ischemic phase is the sigmoid course of the development of intraischemic damage shifted to the left in unwelcome or even dangerous ways?

1. By chronic and acute cardiac illness;
2. By an unfavourable spectrum of effects of the cardioplegic solution;
3. By relatively high temperature during ischemia;
4. By washing out of protective solution during cardiac arrest by non-coronary colateral flow.

We will not discuss these factors at this point, since they need to be gone into separately. Further factors are:

5. High pre-ischemic energy turnover;
6. Lack of equilibrium or steady state during aerobic application of the protective solution;
7. Reduction of the glycogen stores of the heart by a previous ischemic stress;
8. Reduction of the energy-rich phosphates of the heart by a previous ischemic stress;
9. Abnormal initial state of the patient or the donor organism with respect to

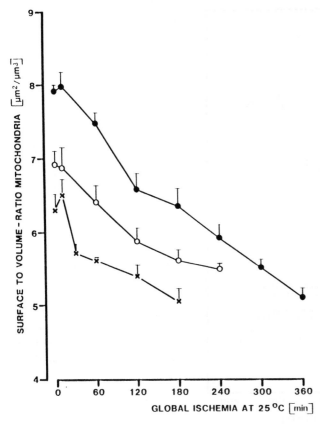

Fig. 4. (a) Surface to volume ratio of mitochondria (S$_v$ratio$_{Mi}$) in the course of global myocardial ischaemia at 25°C following different methods of cardiac arrest, x—x, pure ischaemia; o—o, St. Thomas; o—o, HTK. $\bar{x}$ SEM, n = 6. From Schmiedl et al., 1990 [11].

extracellular or intracellular osmolarity.

As early as 1973, Spieckermann pointed out the significance of energy turnover, which can be influenced by, among other things, the anaesthetic procedure [12]. Figure 5a shows the times up to a drop in phosphocreatine to 3 $\mu M/g_{ww}$ and to a decrease in the ATP level to 4 $\mu M/g_{ww}$ for canine hearts under normothermic conditions, using 8 different types of anaesthetics, and in the case of acute coronary ligature (at the top) and halothane anaesthesia with partial by-pass (at the bottom). Under the latter conditions, the value of 30 min for the ATP time is 6-times greater than that under ketamine anaesthesia, which is 5 min.

The adjustment to a new balance in oxygen consumption following induction of artificial cardiac arrest takes from 3 to 12 min, depending on pre-ischemic turnover, weight of the heart, the condition of the coronary system and the composition of the cardioplegic solution. Bonhoeffer was aware of this problem in 1967, as can be seen from Fig. 5b [1]. The minimal oxygen consumption of

40

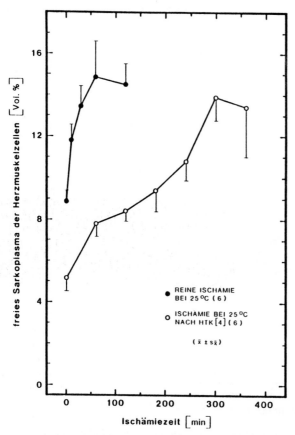

Fig. 4. (b) Development of cellular oedema in the subendocardium of the left ventrical in relation to time; under the condition of the pure global myocardial ischemia and the ischemia after cardioplegia with HTK solution [4]. Results are based on the experiments given in Fig. 8 (see Fig. 8).

the arrested canine heart is, in the steady state, with a favourable case-history, roughly equal to 0.8 ml O_2/min per 100 g. If a steady state is not reached, as in the experiments of Gregg and McKeever employing vagus arrest and potassium chloride arrest, more than twice the values result with a very high scattering. The results of Berglund and co-workers, as well as these of Hoffmeister and co-workers using potassium citrate and potassium chloride, occupy an intermediate position. Thus, it is clear that minimizing the pre-ischemic aerobic energy requirement calls for a previous minimization of the oxygen consumption of the working heart and sufficient time for the aerobic cardioplegic perfusion. Not even the most careful and patient induction of cardioplegia, however, can make the heart or its ischemic tolerance wholly independent of its case history.

Because of the increasing number of surgical operations in cases of cardiac emergencies, sometimes entailing repeated reanimation attempts, and conditions

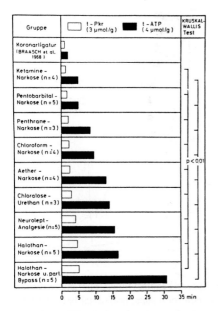
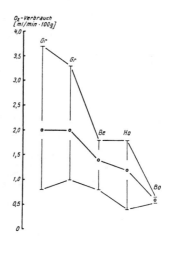

Fig. 5. (a) Values for t-PKr and t-ATP after ligation of the coronaries given by the metabolic changes. These values have been obtained during different kinds of anaesthesia, and after preischemic treatment of the left ventricle by partial bypass and by halothane anaesthesia. From Spieckermann, 1973 [12]. (b) The comparison of the extreme and mean values of arrested dogs' hearts of different teams. Gr = Gregg's group (McKeever et al.): Vagus and potassium chloride arrest; Be = Berglund et al.: potassium citrate arrest. Ho = Hoffmeister et al.: potassium chloride arrest. Bo = Bonhoeffer: heart arrest by withdrawal of sodium and calcium and application of procain. There seems to be a relation between extent of deviation and the amount of the mean values. From Bonhoeffer, 1967 [1].

of donor organisms which are often partly pathological, it seems worthwhile to consider the spectrum of variation in the energy status of the starting points.

In Fig. 6a are depicted the experiments of Conn et al., carried out 32 years ago, which have in no way lost any of their relevance to the problem now before us [6]. A purely ischemic cardiac arrest was induced in 17 non-pretreated and 15 pretreated dogs at 37.5°C and the drop in glycogen and formation of lactate was measured. The pretreatment consisted of infusion with 5 g/kg glucose and 3 U/kg insulin. In this group the glycogen concentration was a factor of 2 higher at the onset of ischemia, and after 2 h, a factor of 4. After the 2 h of ischemia, however, the glycogen stores in the non-pretreated group were almost exhausted. The rapidity of exhaustion of the glycogen as well as of formation of lactate is, in both groups, at least up to 60 min, more or less the same.

In comparison with Fig. 4b, which showed the cellular swelling during ischemia without protection at 25°C, it is obvious that with a physiological starting point and pure ischemia, the glycogen reserves will never be the limiting factor, since at 25°C the cellular swelling is already maximal after 60 min. At

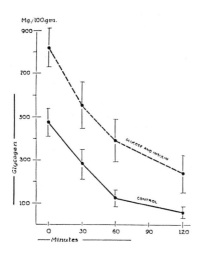
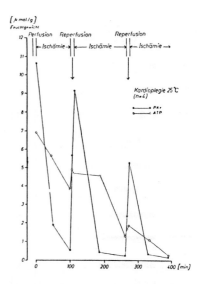

Fig. 6. (a) Mean glycogen concentration in cardiac muscle plotted against time.Upper curve results from hearts treated with glucose and insulin; lower curve, control results; horizontal bars, +2 S.E. of the mean. From Conn et al., 1959 [6]. (b) Behavior of the high-energy phosphates PKr and ATP during ischemia at 25°C and during reperfusion with a cardioplegic solution containing oxygen. From Spieckermann, 1973 [12].

37.5°C after 30 min with the same experimental animal, the dog, even in the untreated group enough glycogen is still present. On the other hand, it must be emphasized that after glycogen reserves are exhausted, no anaerobic energy gains worth mentioning are possible any more; besides which, at lower temperatures and with a good myocardial protection, the glycogen is used up much better than at higher temperatures and with poor protection. The possibility therefore cannot be ruled out that following previous reanimation or longer adrenergic stimulation, the glycogen could become a limiting factor. The replenishing of the glycogen depot of the myocardium needs time, however, even with massive doses of glucose and insulin and potassium when necessary. Conn et al. undertook this pretreatment over periods lasting hours [6].

Preceding ischemic phases decimate not only glycogen reserves but also phosphocreatine and ATP. The first can be rapidly replenished within just a few minutes of aerobic reperfusion, as long as enough ATP is present. Within the framework of replenishment of ATP, a rapid phase which only takes a few minutes must be distinguished from the phase of de novo synthesis, which lasts for days. The rapid phase of ATP regeneration is based on employment of reusable products of decomposition right down to adenosine. Unfortunately, a highly depleted ATP concentration can only be quickly raised by about 20% by this pathway; for instance, a value of 4.0 $\mu M/g_{ww}$ can be improved to approximately 4.8 $\mu M/g_{ww}$. The relevant experiments performed by Spiekermann in 1973 [12] are summarized in Fig. 6b. Canine hearts, arrested by the low-sodium, calcium-free but also buffer-free solution were subjected to three periods of ischemia of 100 min, 150 min and again 150 min at 25°C. The three ischemic periods were interrupted by two aerobic reperfusion phases with the cardioplegic solution, each lasting for 10 min. It is clear that already at 4 $\mu M/g_{ww}$, ATP can only be regenerated to approximately a third of the loss in the rapid regeneration phase. Following the second ischemic phase, the ATP has sunk to a level of under 2 $\mu M/g_{ww}$; thereafter, only a recognizable regeneration of phosphocreatine is possible and no longer any ATP regeneration. The results represent mean values from 4 experiments on dogs. These hearts would, at this time point, certainly also have been no longer revivable. The sharp drop in ATP after 100 min during the second ischemic phase is also interesting. It corresponds to the steep increase in ischemic damage and recovery time.

The starting-point conditions before the induction of cardioplegia and myocardial protection can finally be complicated by an abnormal osmolarity in the extracellular and consequently in the intracellular space. The entire organism and all central organs apparently have at their disposal, under aerobic conditions, several complementary mechanisms which can compensate for deviations from the physiological osmolarity of 290 mosm/l. These include ion pumps, special transport systems and degradation of high molecular weight substances to low molecular weight osmolytes or the reverse. In hypothermia, which, for energetic reasons, is indispensable in organ protection, the compensatory capacity of these regulatory systems is limited. Besides this, they need times of the order of minutes. Water transport due to large differences between osmotic pressures in the extracellular and intracellular space takes place in seconds. Particularly dangerous is a rapid *increase in volume* of the intracellular space, because the interstitium can be thereby compressed and the capillaries closed. For these reasons, the osmolarity of most of the organ protective solutions lies somewhat above the physiological value. If, however, due to inadequate treatment of the donor organism, the sodium concentration should rise to around 190 mM and the overall molarity therefore (due to a corresponding increase in anions) to 400 mosm/l, then there is hardly any chance of saving the organ to be protected. Induction of protection, would, due to osmotic gradients of around 100 mosm/l, corresponding to an osmotic pressure of about 2000 mmHg, cause water to be suddenly forced into the cell. This problem must be neutralized *before* induction of cardioplegia (or *before* conservation of kidney, liver or pancreas), since a general large increase in the osmolarity of the preservative solution would be associated with other disadvantages, for instance, an increase in anaerobic turnover rate and too great a shrinkage of the endothelial barrier.

Finally, let us return to our starting point – to the sigmoid curve of development of ischemic damage and to the interaction between the three central ischemia-dependent processes: development of acidosis, development of cellular oedema and increasing energy deficit.

The above observations should serve to point out that the principal limitations of ischemia (and not, for instance, anoxia) above 0°C for warm-blooded animals

44

cannot be overcome. The time axis of the sigmoid curve of the ischemia-dependent damage – particularly the initial plateau – in very poor conditions, such as hyperthermia, higher turnover rate, predamage, reduced energy reserves and insufficient myocardial protection (cf. Fig. 5a), can be extended by a factor of approximately 200 in optimal conditions, such as preservation temperature, temporary energetic relief, replenishment of all energy reserves, a primarily healthy heart and good myocardial protection.

References

1. Bonnhoeffer K (1967) Der Sauerstoffverbrauch des normo- und hypothermen Hundeherzens vor und während verschiedener Formen des induzierten Herzstillstandes. Basel: Karger.
2. Bretschneider HJ (1961) Sauerstoffbedarf und -versorgung des Herzmuskels. Verh Dtsch Ges Kreislaufforschg 27: 32–59.
3. Bretschneider HJ (1964) Überlebenszeit und Wiederbelebungszeit des Herzens bei Normo- und Hypothermie. Verh Dtsch Ges Kreislaufforschg 30: 11–34.
4. Bretschneider HJ, Hübner G, Knoll D, Lohr B, Nordbeck H, Spieckermann PG (1975) Myocardial resistance and tolerance to ischemia: physiological and biochemical basis. J Cardiovasc Surg 16: 241–260.
5. Bretschneider HJ, Helmchen U, Kehrer G (1988) Nierenprotektion. Klin Wochenschr 66: 817–827.
6. Conn HL, Wood JC, Morales GS (1959) Rate of change in myocardial glycogen and lactic acid following arrest of coronary circulation. Circ Res 7: 721–727.
7. Gebhard MM (1987) Pathophysiologie der globalen Ischämie des Herzens. Z Kardiol 76(Suppl 4): 115–129.
8. Gebhard MM, Gersing E, Brockhoff CJ, Schnabel PhA, Bretschneider HJ (1987) Impedance spectroscopy: a method for surveillance of ischemia tolerance of the heart. Thorac Cardiovasc Surgeon 35: 26–32.
9. Gebhard MM (1990) Myocardial protection and ischemia tolerance of the globally ischemic heart. Thorac Cardiovasc Surgeon 38: 655–659.
10. Gebhard MM (1992) HTK solution in organ protection. In: G Kirste et al., eds. Third Meeting of the HTK-Study group. Wolfgang Pabst-Verlag, in press.
11. Schmiedl A, Schnabel PhA, Mall G, Gebhard MM, Hunneman DH, Richter J, Bretschneider HJ (1990) The surface to volume ratio of mitochondria, a suitable parameter for evaluating mitochondrial swelling. Virchows Arch A Pathol Anat 416: 305–315.
12. Spieckermann PG (1973) Überlebens- und Wiederbelebungszeit des Herzens. In: R Frey, F Kern and O Mayrhofer, eds. Anaesthesiologie und Wiederbelebung Vol. 66. Berlin: Springer-Verlag.

Trauma metabolism and the heart

K. Vyska, K. Minami, R. Körfer, G. Notohamiprodjo and H. Meyer
Herzzentrum NRW, University Hospital Ruhr–University Bochum, Georgstr. 11, D-4970 Bad Oeynhausen, F.R.G.

Introduction

In his animal studies Körfer [1,2] demonstrated that long-term non-pulsatile systemic perfusion by extracorporeal circulation leads in myocardium to the formation of interstitial perivascular oedema without signs of typical hypoxic endothelial injury. In the same study a high number of hypercontractile bands was noted in myocardial cells. Similar observations were noted by both Stemmer et al. [3] and Brody et al. [4] in their analysis of bioptic samples collected intraoperatively in patients undergoing coronary bypass surgery and by Robinson et al. [5] in myocardium of patients who died within 4 days after cardiopulmonary bypass (CPB) application.

Körfer [1,2] postulated that the ischemia does not seem to be a primary cause of this myocardial injury.

It was the aim of the present study to test this hypothesis and to determine whether some changes of myocardial metabolism occurring during the coronary bypass surgery using either pulsatile or non-pulsatile systemic perfusion would be capable of inducing such myocardial injury.

Material and Methods

In this study 20 patients submitted for aortocoronary bypass grafting were examined. None of the patients had valve dysfunction or metabolic disorders in addition to the coronary disease. Patients with unstable angina just before operation were excluded. All patients were hemodynamically stable during surgery without need for inotropic support.

In all patients cardiac medication was stopped 2 days before operation. Patients were premedicated with noctamide and morphine. Anaesthesia was induced by etomidate and fentanyl and maintained by ventilation with oxygen in nitrous oxide with enflurane. Vecuronium was used for muscle relaxation.

Nonpulsatile extracorporeal circulation was performed with a standard Stöckert roller pump. Pulsatile extracorporeal circulation was performed with a double pump system equipped with a pulsatile flow controller. In this system the first pump was inserted between the venous drainage site and the membrane oxygenator and the second between the oxygenator and arterial cannula in the ascending aorta [6].

The blood samples were collected in aortic root and coronary sinus 5 min after cardiopulmonary bypass began (normothermic conditions), at the end of cooling phase before heart fibrillation, at 5 min and at 20 min during rewarming phase after systemic hypothermic myocardial protection. The average duration of cardiopulmonary bypass was 58 min.

We analysed free fatty acid (FFA) plasma concentration, glucose plasma concentration, lactate plasma concentration, oxygen saturation, epinephrine plasma concentration and norepinephrine plasma concentration.

Results and Discussion

The results of free fatty acid determinations are demonstrated in Figs. 1 and 2. The arterial FFA plasma concentrations for both non-pulsatile (NP) and pulsatile (PP) systemic perfusion are presented in Fig. 1.

The arterial–coronary sinus differences related to arterial concentration; the myocardial FFA extraction rates are shown in Fig. 2. It can be seen that although there is a significant blood dilution during the CPB, in all instances arterial FFA concentration is elevated. The FFA extraction rates are seen to be slightly lower than the values observed under physiological conditions [7,8]. The reduced value observed with pulsatile systemic perfusion at the end of cooling phase is expected due to low cardiac temperature. No significant differences were observed between

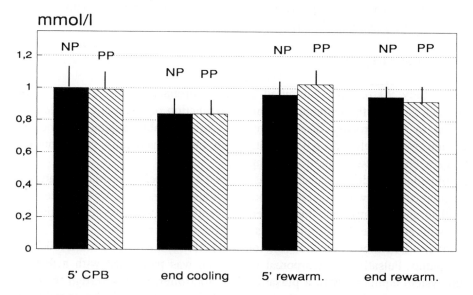

Fig. 1. Arterial free fatty acid (FFA) plasma concentrations detected at four different time intervals during cardiopulmonary bypass (CPB) using nonpulsatile (black bars) or pulsatile (hatched bars) systemic perfusion. Results are presented as means ± SE.

Myocardial FFA Extraction

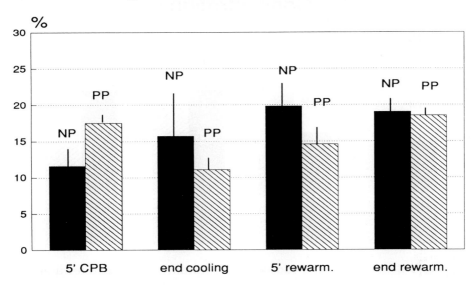

Fig. 2. Myocardial free fatty acid (FFA) extraction observed at four different time intervals during cardiopulmonary bypass (CPB) using nonpulsatile (black bars) or pulsatile (hatched bars) systemic perfusion. Results are presented as means ± SE.

NP and PP either in FFA plasma concentrations or in myocardial FFA extraction rate.

The results of glucose determinations are shown in Figs. 3 and 4. The arterial glucose plasma concentration (Fig. 3) observed during cooling phase is seen to correspond to physiological values. During the rewarming phase the arterial glucose plasma concentration is increased, probably as a consequence of mobilisation of glucose from intracellular stores.

When compared to basic conditions, glucose extraction seems to be reduced (under basic conditions a value of 10% is expected). If it is, however, considered that during CPB the plasma is diluted to 50% of its physiological value, it appears that the glucose uptake is only slightly reduced under CPB conditions. In our opinion, this slight reduction of glucose uptake reflects reduced myocardial energy requirements and reduced myocardial work of vented heart. In this connection, however, insulin resistance mediated by high levels of stress hormones should be discussed as well. There were no significant differences between NP and PP either in arterial glucose plasma concentration or in glucose extraction.

The results of lactate plasma concentrations are shown in Figs. 5 and 6. As demonstrated in Fig. 6, in both pulsatile and non-pulsatile systemic perfusion, there is slight lactate uptake in the early part of the cooling phase and no uptake or release at the end of cooling phase. The slight release of lactate was observed throughout the rewarming phase. This might be the consequence of slight

Arterial Glucose Plasma Concentration

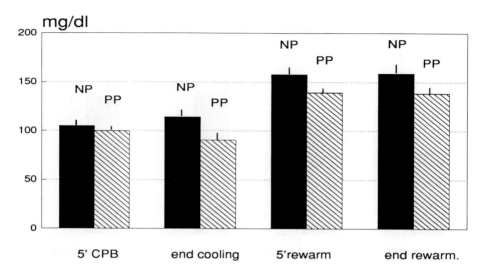

Fig. 3. Arterial glucose plasma concentrations detected at four different time intervals during cardiopulmonary bypass (CPB) using nonpulsatile (black bars) or pulsatile (hatched bars) systemic perfusion. Results are presented as means ± SE.

Myocardial Glucose Extraction

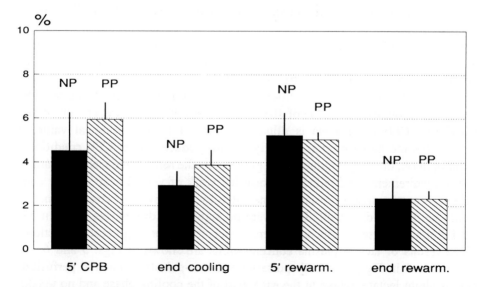

Fig. 4. Myocardial glucose extraction observed at four different time intervals during cardiopulmonary bypass (CPB) using nonpulsatile (black bars) or pulsatile (hatched bars) systemic perfusion. Results are presented as means ± SE.

Arterial Lactate Plasma Concentration

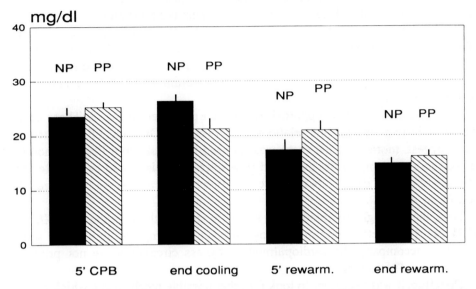

Fig. 5. Arterial lactate plasma concentrations detected at four different time intervals during cardiopulmonary bypass (CPB) using nonpulsatile (black bars) or pulsatile (hatched bars) systemic perfusion. Results are presented as means ± SE.

(Arterio -Coronary Sinus) Difference of Lactate Plasma Concentrations

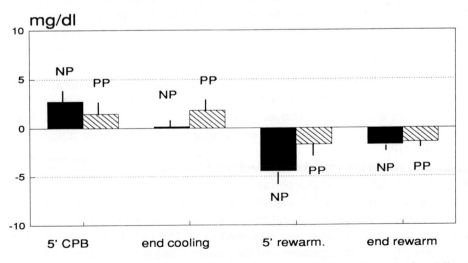

Fig. 6. Arterio–coronary sinus difference of lactate plasma concentrations observed at four different time intervals during cardiopulmonary bypass (CPB) using nonpulsatile (black bars) or pulsatile (hatched bars) systemic perfusion. Results are presented as means ± SE.

ischemia probably existing during the surgery. No significant differences were observed between NP and PP either in lactate plasma concentrations or in arterial-coronary sinus difference of lactate plasma concentrations.

The oxygen extraction is shown in Fig. 7. In this figure, it can be seen that in all examined time intervals the oxygen extraction was significantly lower than the values observed under physiological conditions. This finding demonstrates the reduced energy requirements of vented myocardium and indicates sufficient perfusion during the surgery.

This conclusion is also supported by the data presented in Fig. 8. These data, which indicate a straight-line relationship between $AVDO_2$ and FFA extraction rate, suggest, moreover, that there was no need to switch from FFA to another energy source in any of the examined time intervals (this would be expected in the case of oxygen deficit). No significant differences were observed between NP and PP in $AVDO_2$.

Thus, the findings presented so far seems to support the hypothesis of Körfer [1,2] that the structural and morphological changes in myocardium which were found to accompany the cardiopulmonary bypass circulation are not primary consequences of ischemia.

Therefore, it was necessary to look for other possible mechanisms which might lead to myocardial injury described above. For this, we analysed the arterial and coronary sinus plasma concentrations of epinephrine and norepinephrine as well.

Figure 9 shows arterial epinephrine concentrations. For all examined time intervals a significantly higher ($p < 0.01$) arterial epinephrine concentration was found with nonpulsatile when compared to pulsatile systemic perfusion and physiological values (the physiological value of plasma epinephrine concentration was estimated to be 15 pg/ml, from the data reported by Ganong [9] for normal persons and the plasma dilution factor detected during CPB). The increase of arterial epinephrine concentration with NP was expected, since as demonstrated by Minami et al. [6] the absence of pulse amplitude with nonpulsatile perfusion leads via baroreceptors to increase of sympathetic tone.

Also arterio-coronary sinus differences of epinephrine plasma concentrations in all examined time intervals were found to be significantly higher ($p < 0.01$) than the values observed with nonpulsatile systemic perfusion (see Fig. 10). This indicates higher storage or catabolic degradation of epinephrine in myocardial tissue with NP.

Figure 11 shows the arterial norepinephrine plasma concentrations observed in this study. The arterial norepinephrine concentration increased during cardiopulmonary bypass with both NP and PP. The initial values were comparable to values observed under physiological conditions (the physiological value of plasma norepinephrine concentration was estimated to be 150 pg/ml, the data reported by Ganong [9] for normal persons and the plasma dilution factor detected during CPB). In contrast to PP with NP the circulating levels of norepinephrine in coronary sinus were significantly higher than those detected in arterial plasma. Correspondingly, as demonstrated in Fig. 12, the arterio-coronary sinus

AVDO$_2$

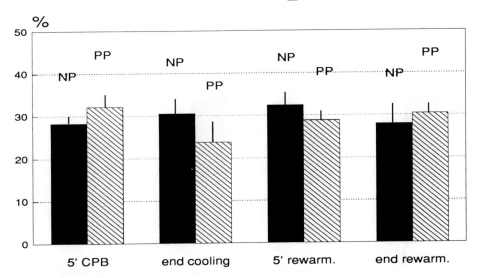

Fig. 7. Myocardial oxygen extraction observed at four different time intervals during cardiopulmonary bypass (CPB) using nonpulsatile (black bars) or pulsatile (hatched bars) systemic perfusion. Results are presented as means ± SE.

(Arterio-Coronary Sinus) Difference of FFA Plasma Concentrations vs AVDO2

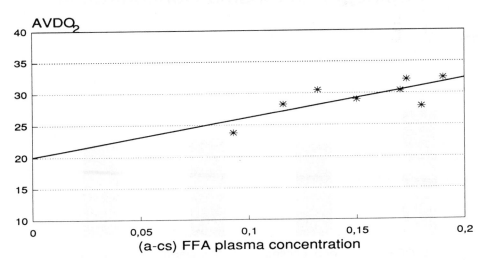

Fig. 8. Average values of arterio-coronary sinus differences of free fatty acid (FFA) plasma concentrations detected at four different time intervals during cardiopulmonary bypass (CPB) using either NP or PP are plotted against average values of myocardial oxygen extraction.

52

Arterial Epinephrine Plasma Concentration

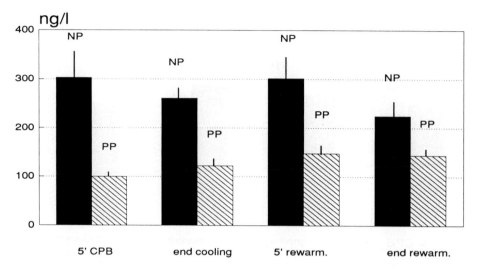

Fig. 9. Arterial epinephrine plasma concentrations detected at four different time intervals during cardiopulmonary bypass (CPB) using nonpulsatile (black bars) or pulsatile (hatched bars) systemic perfusion. Results are presented as means ± SE.

(Arterio - Coronary Sinus) Difference of Epinephrine Plasma Concentrations

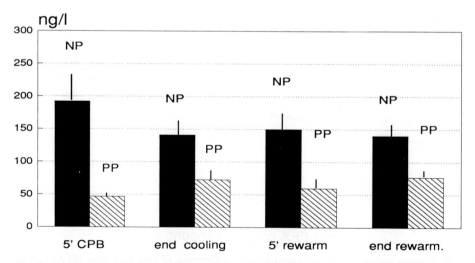

Fig. 10. Arterio-coronary sinus difference of epinephrine plasma concentrations observed at four different time intervals during cardiopulmonary bypass (CPB) using nonpulsatile (black bars) or pulsatile (hatched bars) systemic perfusion. Results are presented as means ± SE.

Arterial Norepinephrine Plasma Concentration

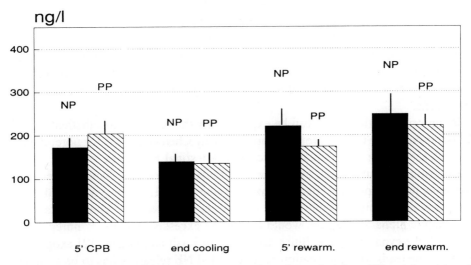

Fig. 11. Arterial norepinephrine plasma concentrations detected at four different time intervals during cardiopulmonary bypass (CPB) using nonpulsatile (black bars) or pulsatile (hatched bars) systemic perfusion. Results are presented as means ± SE.

(Arterio - Coronary Sinus) Difference of Norepinephrine Plasma Concentrations

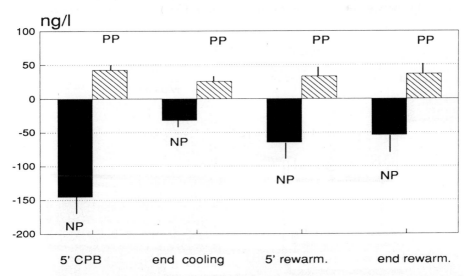

Fig. 12. Arterio-coronary sinus difference of norepinephrine plasma concentrations observed at four different time intervals during cardiopulmonary bypass (CPB) using nonpulsatile (black bars) or pulsatile (hatched bars) systemic perfusion. Results are presented as means ± SE.

54

differences observed with NP were negative. These results, which were statistically significant ($p < 0.01$), indicate that there was a significant release of norepinephrine into coronary sinus with nonpulsatile perfusion. The release of norepinephrine into coronary sinus detected with nonpulsatile systemic perfusion was not detected with pulsatile systemic perfusion either in this study or by Yamaguchi et al. [10] under physiological conditions.

In this connection, the question arose why at comparable norepinephrine arterial concentration NE is released into coronary sinus with nonpulsatile perfusion, whereas it is extracted with pulsatile systemic perfusion or under basal conditions.

In our opinion, this effect can be explained by the use of a hypothetical model for norepinephrine release proposed originally by Chen et al. [11] for norepinephrine release during autoregulatory escape in intestinal resistance vessels.

According to this model, sympathetic stimulation causes enhanced release of norepinephrine from the nerve terminal (see Fig. 13). Presynaptic alpha-2 receptors enable norepinephrine to inhibit its own release. The blockade of presynaptic alpha-2 receptors would lead to an excessive release of norepinephrine into the synaptic space. Since according to Raab and Gigee [12] exogenous epinephrine leads to augmentation of myocardial NE release it has to be assumed that the high epinephrine plasma concentrations accompanied by high epinephrine extraction influence the presynaptic alpha-2 receptors and thus inhibit the reuptake of norepinephrine in presynaptic endings.

If this mechanism is applied to our observations with nonpulsatile perfusion indicating high epinephrine plasma concentrations, high epinephrine extraction, increased norepinephrine release into coronary sinus and a straight-line relationship between arterio–coronary sinus difference of epinephrine and

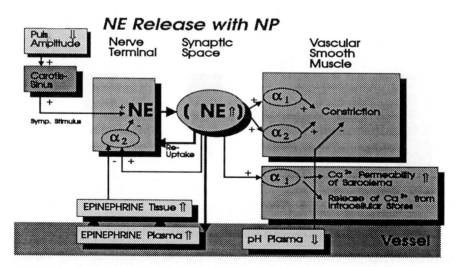

Fig. 13. Hypothetical model for control mechanism which leads to norepinephrine release into coronary sinus in the case of nonpulsatile systemic perfusion.

norepinephrine plasma concentrations (see Fig. 14), then it has to be expected that under conditions of nonpulsatile systemic perfusion there is an excessive accumulation of norepinephrine in synaptic space, which leads to a high concentration gradient between synaptic space and plasma and thus to the observed release of norepinephrine into plasma and finally into coronary sinus.

If in this connection it is considered that according to Downing et al. [13] and Chen et al. [14] the excessive accumulation of endogenously released norepinephrine in the synaptic space is capable of inducing myocardial injury in humans [15–17] then it becomes evident that nonpulsatile systemic perfusion might cause myocardial injury.

With respect to the pathogenetic mechanisms of norepinephrine-induced myocardial injury, several possibilities were discussed in the past.

Simons and Downing [18], Tsutsui et al. [19] and Nishigaki et al. [20] have demonstrated that alpha-adrenergic receptors can be found at high concentrations along coronary arteries and at lower concentrations along the coronary veins and that at a given norepinephrine concentration the relative constriction of venules is comparable to that of arterioles. This means that the excessive accumulation of NE in synaptic space observed in our study would lead to a reduction of the cross-section in both arterial and venous system. The reduction of cross-section in the venous part of circulation would not reduce the perfusion but it could lead to a significant increase of capillary pressure.

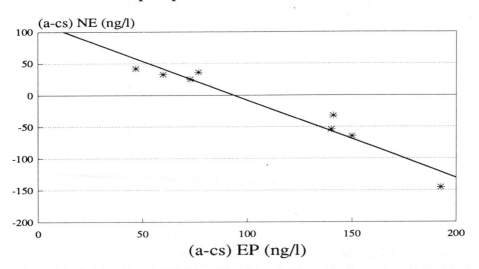

(a-cs) Epinephrine vs (a-cs) Norepinephrine Plasma Concentration

Fig. 14. Average values of arterio–coronary sinus differences of norepinephrine plasma concentrations detected at different time intervals during cardiopulmonary bypass (CPB) using either NP or PP are plotted against arterio–coronary sinus differences of epinephrine plasma concentrations.

56

The increased capillary pressure would lead to an increase of filtration pressure and might explain the observed perivascular oedema in human heart observed with cardiopulmonary bypass circulation.

On the other hand, in their animal experiments Simons and Downing demonstrated [18] that the extensive myocardial alpha-1 receptor stimulation might lead to an increase of extracellular Ca^{2+} influx through a Ca^{2+} channel in the plasma membrane and to a release of intracellularly bound Ca^{2+}. Consequently, it has to be expected that the excessive accumulation of endogenously released norepinephrine in synaptic space with nonpulsatile perfusion might lead to an overload of myocardial cells with Ca^{2+}. This would explain the observed hypercontractile bands observed in myocardium after long-term nonpulsatile perfusion.

The analysis presented so far thus suggests that under conditions of cardiopulmonary bypass circulation with nonpulsatile systemic perfusion the increased sympathetic tone induced via carotis sinus baroreceptors by the absence of blood pressure pulsations may lead to: (i) norepinephrine overload of postganglionic synapsis; and so (ii) to venoconstriction; (iii) increased capillary pressure; (iv) increased fluid filtration into extravascular space; and (v) overloading of cardiac tissue with Ca^{2+}; and thus to myocardial injury even in the absence of ischemia.

References

1. Körfer R (1979) Habilitationsschrift. Universität Düsseldorf.
2. Körfer R, Steven W, Frenzel H, Arnold G (1980) ESAO Proc VII: 294.
3. Stemmer KA, Ikonjo J, Aronow WS, Thilbaut W, et al. (1975) J Thorac Cardiovasc Surg 70: 666.
4. Brody WR, Reitz BA, Andrews MJ, Roberts WC, et al. (1975) J Thorac Cardiovasc Surg 70: 1073.
5. Robinson MJ, Lam R, Morales AR (1977) Am J Clin Path 68: 721.
6. Minami K, Körner M, Vyska K, Kleesiek K, et al. (1990) J Thorac Cardiovasc Surg 99: 82-91.
7. Vyska K, Meyer W, Stremmel W, Notohamiprodjo G (1991) Circ Res 69: 857-870.
8. Vyska K, Machulla HJ, Stremmel W, Fassbender D (1988) Circulation 78: 1218-1223.
9. Ganong WF (1977) Review of Medical Physiology. 9th Edition Los Altos, CA: Lange Medical Publications, 159.
10. Yamaguchi N, de Chaplain J, Nadenau R (1975) Circ Res 86: 662-668.
11. Chen LQ, Riedel GL, Shepherd AP (1991) Am J Physiol 260: (Heart Circ Physiol 29) H400-H408.
12. Raab W, Gigee W (1955) Circ Res 3: 553-558.
13. Downing SE, Chen V (1985) J Mol Cell Cardiol 17: 377-387.
14. Chen V, Downing SE (1990) Am J Physiol 258; (Heart Circ Physiol 27) H101-H106.
15. Kline IK (1961) Am J Pathol 38: 539-557.
16. Reichenbach DD, Benditt EP (1970) Human Pathol 1: 125-150.
17. Szakacs JE, Cannon I (1958) Am J Clin Pathol 30: 425-434.
18. Simons M, Downing SE (1985) Am Heart J 109: 297-304.
19. Tsutsui H, Tomoike H, Nakamura M (1990) Am J Physiol 259; (Heart Circ Physiol 28) H1343-1350.
20. Nishigaki K, Faber JE, Ohyanagi M (1991) Am J Physiol 260; (Heart Circ Physiol 29) H1655-H1666.

Pulsatile and non-pulsatile perfusion

Kenneth M. Taylor
Royal Postgraduate Medical School, Hammersmith Hospital, London, U.K.

Introduction

As overall mortality in cardiac surgery has reduced, research effort has increasingly been directed towards reducing morbidity. In this era of 'refinement' in cardiac surgery techniques, the role of cardiopulmonary bypass (CPB) in inducing organ dysfunction during and after surgery has been identified as a major area of interest.

The pathophysiology of CPB is considered to involve at least two major factors: (1) altered blood flow delivery – low flow, low pressure, non-pulsatile; (2) blood cell activation – microembolism, and a systemic inflammatory response.

This chapter concentrates on blood flow during CPB, focussing particularly on the issue of pulsatile and non-pulsatile perfusion, firstly as it relates to haemodynamics in general and secondly as it might affect splanchnic perfusion.

Flow rates during cardiopulmonary bypass

During CPB, the body's ability to vary cardiac output to match overall energy demands is temporarily lost. The artificial bypass pump delivers whatever flow rate is set by the perfusionist. Although physiologic blood flow rates are approximately 3–3.2 $l/m^2/min$, flow rates on CPB are customarily set at 2.2–2.4 $l/m^2/min$ [1–3]. This moderate flow perfusion represents a degree of compromise because higher flows are believed to be associated with increased blood cell trauma. Although higher flows have recently been used in infants on extracorporeal membrane oxygenation (ECMO) [4], and have also been used experimentally [5–7], there is no move to advocate higher flow rates for routine CPB.

Instead, the use of moderate hypothermia during CPB has encouraged some workers to reduce CPB flow rates even further. Tissue oxygen requirements fall progressively with reductions in temperature. Whole body oxygen consumption has been shown to fall from around 120 $ml/m^2/min$ at 37°C to 33 $ml/m^2/min$ at 20°C where perfusion flow is maintained at 2.4 $l/m^2/min$. Studies have shown that flow rates may safely be reduced to 1.6 $l/m^2/min$ at core temperatures of 28°C and that at 20°C flow rates of 1.2 $l/m^2/min$ are still adequate, though flow reserve is limited [8]. Another argument used in favour of low-flow perfusion relates to myocardial protection. Noncoronary collateral blood flow limits the efficacy of cold cardioplegic techniques. Pump flow rates reduced to 1.5 $l/m^2/min$ produce a 60% reduction in noncoronary collateral flows.

Vasoconstriction during cardiopulmonary bypass

From the earliest days of open-heart surgery, it has been recognised that the use of conventional non-pulsatile perfusion is associated with significant and progressive systemic vasoconstriction.

The pathologic consequences of vasoconstriction include (1) reduced perfusion of peripheral organs, and (2) increased left ventricular work.

With a small rise in vascular resistance, and normal myocardial function, there will be an increase in myocardial performance and ventricular work in accordance with the Starling curve [9]. However, large increases in peripheral resistance may impose an excessive afterload on the left ventricle, with eventual reduction in cardiac pumping efficiency and fall in output. In patients whose ventricular function is already compromised and whose reserve is limited, small rises in vascular resistance may result in cardiac decompensation. Once vasoconstriction has become established, a vicious circle may develop, with a reduced cardiac output leading to peripheral circulatory inadequacy and the consequent release of vasoconstrictor substances that further raise vascular resistance and thereby diminish cardiac output [10].

The early days of cardiac surgery were marked by a frequent incidence of low-cardiac-output syndromes. Though preservation techniques have improved the contractility of the recovering myocardium, it is logical that maintenance of vascular resistance at normal levels would lead to better cardiac performance in the recovery period. Subsequent studies have shown that where high peripheral vascular resistance levels are reduced following cardiac surgery (using such vasodilator techniques as epidural anaesthesia and sodium nitroprusside), a significant increase in cardiac performance is seen [11,12].

Vasoconstrictor mechanisms during cardiac surgery

A number of causes have been proposed to explain the vasoconstrictive response to open-heart surgery. These include (1) catecholamine release, (2) activation of the renin-angiotensin system, (3) increased secretion of vasopressin (ADH), and (4) local tissue vasoconstrictor agents (e.g. thromboxane A_2).

A number of reports have indicated that catecholamine secretion is increased during and after open-heart surgery. This may be related to the use of hypothermia, but may also be a response to the altered perfusion associated with the use of nonpulsatile flow. Both vasopressin (ADH) and renin-angiotensin activation have been related to nonpulsatile perfusion. Lack of pulsatility in the arterial circulation appears to trigger both of these important vasoconstrictor mechanisms. The speed of response of vasopressin release appears higher than does that of renin-angiotensin activation, which has been extensively studied [13–15]. The potential role of thromboxane A_2 in the vasoconstrictive response to cardiac surgery has only recently emerged [16]. Although the increased thromboxane production may be a result of nonpulsatile perfusion, the role of platelet activation (a major consequence of extracorporeal circulation) may be more important.

Renin-angiotensin activation during cardiac surgery

It has been known for many years that loss of pulsation in the renal arteries, while mean flow and pressure are maintained, increases the release of renin [17,18]. The end product of renin-angiotensin activation is the powerful vasoconstrictor angiotensin II. Marked rises in plasma angiotensin II have been demonstrated both during and after cardiac surgical procedures [13-15]. In addition to its vasoconstrictive action, angiotensin II has been shown to produce subendocardial ischemia. There is a significant correlation between the rise in angiotensin II levels and the increased vascular resistance index during cardiac surgery. The important role of angiotensin II in postoperative haemodynamics may be seen when elevated angiotensin II levels are rapidly reduced using a specific angiotensin I to angiotensin II converting enzyme inhibitor. A highly significant fall in vascular resistance levels is seen with a simultaneous increase in cardiac index [19] (Fig. 1).

In addition to the above vasoconstrictor mechanisms, recent studies have suggested that local vascular endothelium may respond to non-pulsatile blood flow by promoting a local vasoconstrictive response. Excess production of thromboxane A_2 has been described [16], and most recently it has been shown that non-pulsatile flow significantly reduces endothelial release of endothelial-derived relaxant-factor (EDRF) [20].

Haemodynamic effects of pulsatile perfusion during CPB

It is not generally appreciated that the principal argument for the benefit of pulsatile perfusion in cardiac surgery is related to its haemodynamic effects. Many investigators have jumped straight to studies of vital organ function (e.g. kidney, lung, brain and liver) without first demonstrating that the primary haemodynamic effects had been achieved. Only when such primary haemo-dynamic effects are achieved may one expect to find any secondary vital organ improvements.

The primary effect of pulsatile perfusion is the prevention of the vasoconstric-tion associated with non-pulsatile flow. Such a vasoconstrictive response to non-pulsatile flow has been recognised for many years and has been a recurrent finding in experimental and clinical studies [22-26].

Maintenance of normal levels of peripheral vascular resistance throughout CPB also confers a secondary haemodynamic benefit in that, at the end of the period of CPB, the left ventricle is not exposed to any increased afterload. Left ventricular function, workload, and cardiac output are, therefore, optimised [27].

These two important haemodynamic benefits of pulsatile perfusion are of particular importance in patients with pre-existing compromised left ventricular

60

function. Clinical studies have reported significant reductions in haemodynamic morbidity and mortality associated with the use of pulsatile perfusion [26,28].

Two important points must be made in relation to the practical application of pulsatile CPB.

(1) *Variability in pulsatile blood flow delivered* Few studies have actually characterised the nature of the pulsatile flow delivered. Different pulsatile pump systems generate different pulsatile wave forms (Figs. 2 and 3). The need to

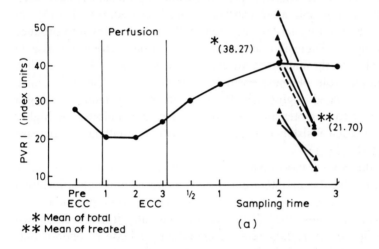

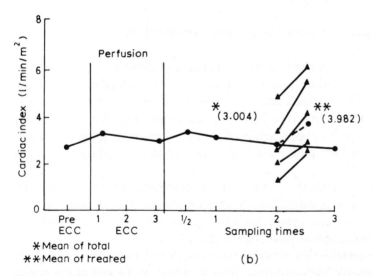

Fig. 1. (a) Effect of angiotensin-converting enzyme inhibition (drug SQ 14225) on peripheral vascular resistance index (PVRI) levels following non-pulsatile cardiopulmonary bypass. (Reprinted with permission from Ref. 19). (b) Effect of angiotensin-converting enzyme inhibition (drug SQ 14225) on peripheral vascular resistance index (PVRI) levels following non-pulsatile cardiopulmonary bypass. (Reprinted with permission from Ref. 19).

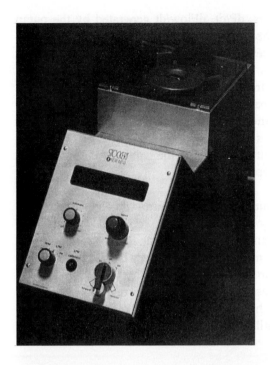

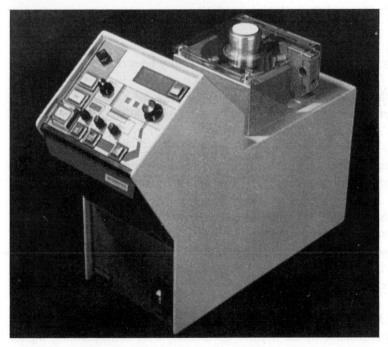

Fig. 2. Two modified roller pump systems (above) Stockert and (below) Sarns suitable for clinical pulsatile perfusion.

provide clear data on flows, pressures, dP/dt, dFlow/dt generated by the pump itself, together with similar data on the wave forms generated within the patient's circulation has been emphasised by several investigators [29,30]. Actual Fourier analysis of pulsatile wave forms has recently been advocated by Sohma et al. [31]. Other components of the CPB circuit may significantly modify the pulsatile flow delivered to the patient. In particular, membrane oxygenators, arterial cannulas and, to a lesser extent, arterial line filters may exert a significant damping effect [32] (Fig. 3). Studies that purport to show change or lack of change in vital organ function without first defining the nature of their delivered pulsatile flow are impossible to interpret.

(2) *Variability in anaesthetic techniques* Many literature studies in the pulsatile/non-pulsatile flow controversy give little or no details of anaesthetic techniques used. High-dose narcotic anaesthesia may block the normal endocrine stress responses. B-blocker therapy may modify renin release and subsequent angiotensin activation. Most importantly, an anaesthetic technique that is vasodilatory may reduce peripheral vascular resistance to less than 50% of normal values during the period of CPB. In the presence of a low PVRI, pulsatile pump systems will not produce the pulsatile flow patterns seen at normal levels of vascular resistance.

Pulsatile perfusion and the splenic circulation

Several recent reviews have reported gastro-intestinal complications following cardiac surgery in 0.6–2.0% of patients, with mortality rates of between 12% and 67% [33–35]. The commonest G-I complication appears to be G-I bleeding, followed by cholecystitis and pancreatitis (Desai and Ohri [37]). Sub-clinical evidence of gut mucosal ischaemia has been reported in 50% of patients in Fiddian-Green's series [36].

White blood cell activation (probably initially through contact activation of Factor XII) may induce an acute inflammatory response and may produce splanchnic microembolism. Vasoconstriction and splanchnic ischaemia may also be important. Hypoperfusion consequent upon the vasoconstriction of non-pulsatile flow has recently been implicated as a possible aetiological factor in gut ischaemia during cardiac surgery [37].

Is there any evidence that splanchnic perfusion may have been optimised by the use of pulsatile CPB?

Mathie et al. [38] have reported that pulsatile perfusion maintains significantly lower vascular resistance in the hepatic circulation, with corresponding higher liver blood flow, when compared with non-pulsatile perfusion. Pancreatic iso-amylase levels were shown by Desai and Ohri [37] to be significantly lower with pulsatile perfusion, confirming earlier work by Murray et al. [39] using the

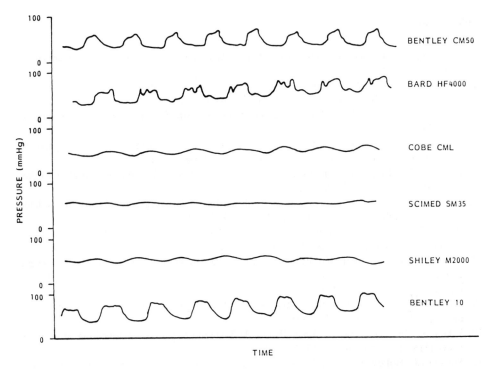

Fig. 3. Modification of pulsatile wave forms by hollow-fibre oxygenators (Bentley CM50 and Bard H4000), flat sheet membrane oxygenators (Cobe CML, Scimed 5M 35 and Shiley M 2000) compared to control (Bentley 10 bubble oxygenator). (Reprinted with permission from Ref. 30).

amylase creatinine clearance ratio (ACCR). Indirect evidence of reduced G-I complications with pulsatile flow was reported recently by Desai et al. [40], who found a 0.18% incidence in pulsed patients compared to a 0.76% incidence in non-pulsed patients. This was a retrospective study of over 2,000 patients. A prospective, randomised clinical study is in progress in the author's unit, studying intramucosal pH and pO_2 levels during pulsatile and non-pulsatile CPB, using the Tonomitor (Tonometrics, Bethesda, MD) described previously by Fiddian-Green and Baker [36].

Whatever else, it is clear that the effects of CPB on the splanchnic circulation require considerable further study. Although the incidence of overt G-I complications may be relatively low, such complications often carry a substantial mortality. It seems certain that the incidence of sub-clinical gut dysfunction is considerable, and that better understanding of the mechanisms of injury will lead to improved methods of prevention and treatment. Pulsatile perfusion has been shown to optimise haemodynamics in the circulation in general. It seems reasonable to expect that it might also be shown to optimise splanchnic perfusion in particular.

64

References

1. Taylor KM (1990) The haemodynamics of cardiopulmonary bypass. Sem Thorac Cardiovasc Surg 2: 300-312.
2. Vasko JS, Dearing JP (1972) Techniques of cardiopulmonary perfusion. In: JC Norman, ed. Cardiac Surgery. New York, NY, Appleton-Century-Crofts.
3. Tarhan S, Moffitt EA (1971) Anaesthesia and supportive care during and after cardiac surgery. Ann Thorac Surg 11: 64-89.
4. Bartlett RH, Andrews AF, Toomasian JM, et al. (1982) Extracorporeal membrane oxygenation (ECMO) for newborn respiratory failure; 45 cases. Surgery 92: 425-433.
5. Boucher JK, Rudy LW, Edmunds LH (1974) Organ blood flow during pulsatile cardio-pulmonary bypass. J Appl Physiol 36: 86-90.
6. Harken AH (1975) The influence of pulsatile perfusion on oxygen uptake by the isolated canine hind limb. J Thorac Cardiovasc Surg 70: 237-241.
7. Rudy LW, Heymann MA, Edmunds LH (1973) Distribution of systemic blood flow during cardiopulmonary bypass. J Appl Physiol 34: 194-200.
8. Fox LS, Blackstone EH, Kirklin JW, et al. (1982) Relationship of whole body oxygen consumption to perfusion flow rate during hypothermic cardiopulmonary bypass. J Thorac Cardiovasc Surg 83: 239-248.
9. Sonnenblick EH, Downing SE (1963) Afterload as a primary determinant of ventricular performance. Am J Physiol 204: 604-608.
10. Estafanous FG, Tarazi RC, Viljoen JF (1973) Systemic hypertension following myocardial revascularisation. Am Heart J 85: 732-738.
11. Stinson EB, Holloway EL, Derby GC, et al. (1977) Control of myocardial performance early after open-heart operations by vasodilator treatment. J Thorac Cardiovasc Surg 73: 523-538.
12. Taylor KM, Casals J, Morton JJ, et al. (1979) The haemodynamic effects of angiotensin blockade after cardiopulmonary bypass. Br Heart J 41: 380.
13. Taylor KM, Bain WH, Russell M, et al. (1979) Peripheral vascular resistance and angiotensin II levels during pulsatile and non-pulsatile cardiopulmonary bypass. Thorax 34: 594-598.
14. Taylor KM, Casals J, Morton JJ, et al. (1979) The haemodynamic effects of angiotensin blockade after cardiopulmonary bypass. Br Heart J 41: 380.
15. Taylor KM, Bain WH, Morton JJ, et al. (1980) The role of angiotensin II in the development of peripheral vasoconstriction during open-heart surgery. Am Heart J 100: 935-937.
16. Watkins DM, Peterson MB, Kong DL, et al. (1982) Thromboxane and prostacyclin changes during cardiopulmonary bypass with and without pulsatile flow. J Thorac Cardiovasc Surg 84: 250-256.
17. Kohlstaedt KG, Page IH (1940) The liberation of renin by perfusion of kidneys following reduction of pulse pressure. J Exp Med 72: 201-205.
18. Many M, Soroff HS, Birtwell WC, et al. (1967) The physiological role of pulsatile and non-pulsatile blood flow. II: Effects on renal function. Arch Surg 95: 762-766.
19. Taylor KM, Casals JG, Brown JJ, et al. (1980) Haemodynamic effects of SQ14225 after cardiopulmonary bypass. Cardiovasc Res 14: 199-205.
20. Pohl U, Busse R, Kuon E, Bassenge E (1986) Pulsatile perfusion stimulates the release of endothelial autacoids. J Appl Card 1: 215-235.
21. Jacobs LA, Klopp EH, Seamone W, et al. (1969) Improved organ function during cardiopul-monary bypass with a roller pump modified to deliver pulsatile flow. J Thorac Cardiovasc Surg 58: 703-712.
22. Takeda J (1960) Experimental study of peripheral circulation during extracorporeal circulation. Arch Jpn Chir 29: 1407-1412.

23. Nakayama K, Tamiya T, Yamamoto K (1963) High amplitude pulsatile pump in extracorporeal circulation with particular reference to haemodynamics. Surgery 54: 798–802.

24. Mendelbaum I, Burns WH (1965) Pulsatile and non-pulsatile blood flow. J Am Med Assoc 191: 121–123.

25. Trinkle JK, Helton NE, Wood RC (1969) Metabolic comparison of a new pulsatile pump and a roller pump for cardiopulmonary bypass. J Thorac Cardiovasc Surg 58: 562–566.

26. Bregman D, Bowman FO, Parodi EN, et al. (1977) An improved method of myocardial protection with pulsation during cardiopulmonary bypass. Circulation (suppl 2); 56: 157–160.

27. Maddoux G, Pappas G, Jenkins M, et al. (1976) Effect of pulsatile and nonpulsatile flow during cardiopulmonary bypass on left ventricular ejection fraction early after aortocoronary bypass surgery. Am J Cardiol 37: 1000–1004.

28. Taylor KM (1981) Why pulsatile flow during cardiopulmonary bypass? In: DB Longmore, ed. Towards Safer Cardiac Surgery. Lancaster: MTP 481–500.

29. Wright G (1988) The hydraulic power outputs of pulsatile and nonpulsatile cardiopulmonary bypass pumps. Perfusion 3: 251–262.

30. Gourlay T, Gibbons W, Taylor KM (1987) Pulsatile flow compatibility of a group of membrane oxygenators. Perfusion 2: 115–126.

31. Sohma A, Ohga K, Oka T, et al. (1989) Quantitative analysis of the effect of pulsatile flow on vascular resistance. Perfusion 4: 213–221.

32. Wright G (1989) Factors affecting the pulsatile hydraulic power output of the Stockert roller pump. Perfusion 4: 187–195.

33. Welling RE, Rath R, Albers JE, Glaser RS (1986) Gastrointestinal complications after cardiac surgery. Arch Surg 121: 1178–1180.

34. Leitman MI, Paull DE, Barie PS, et al. (1987) Intra-abdominal complications of cardiopulmonary bypass operations. Surg Gynaecol Obstet 165: 251–254.

35. Krasna MJ, Francbaum L, Trooskin SZ, et al. (1988) Gastrointestinal complications after cardiac surgery. Surgery 104: 773–780.

36. Fiddian-Green RG, Baker S (1987) The predictive value of measurements of pH in the wall of the stomach for complications after cardiac surgery: a comparison with other forms of monitoring. Crit Care Med 15: 153–156.

37. Desai JB, Ohri SK (1990) Review article – Gastrointestinal damage following cardiopulmonary bypass. Perfusion 5: 161–168.

38. Mathie RT, Desai JB, Taylor KM, et al. (1986) The effect of normothermic cardiopulmonary bypass on hepatic blood flow in the dog. Perfusion 1: 245–253.

39. Murray WR, Mittra S, Mittra D, et al. (1982) The amylase creatinine clearance ratio following cardiopulmonary bypass. J Thorac Cardiovasc Surg 82: 248–253.

40. Desai J, Ohri SK, Roussak J, et al. (in press) Pulsatile flow and the incidence of gastrointestinal complications after cardiopulmonary bypass. Eur J Cardiothor Surg.

Effects of pulsatile perfusion on perioperative morbidity and mortality in high-risk patients

K. Minami, W. Dramburg, G. Notohamiprodjo and R. Körfer

Department of Thoracic and Cardiovascular Surgery, Heart Center North Rhine–Westphalia, University of Bochum, 4970 Bad Oeynhausen, Georgstrasse 11, F.R.G.

Introduction

Extracorporeal circulation (ECC) with pulsatile perfusion (PP) has proved to be more favourable for the total organism as well as for individual organ systems than nonpulsatile perfusion (NP) regarding arterial circulation, coronary perfusion and micro- and lymph circulation [1–4].

Although the hemodynamic advantages of pulsatile perfusion could be demonstrated in several experimental [4–6] and clinical studies [7–11], routine use of the PP during cardiac procedures has been hampered by the lack of technologically satisfactory pulsatile pump systems and a significant increase in postoperative hemolysis.

One of the aims of this retrospective study is to demonstrate improvement of the morbidity and mortality in high-risk patients undergoing cardiac operation by using pulsatile ECC. The other aim is to show elimination of blood damage using a recently developed double pump system for pulsatile perfusion.

Patients and Methods

One hundred and seventy-five patients who underwent cardiac operation with ECC longer than 120 min were studied in two groups. In 88 patients (group A) nonpulsatile perfusion was used and in 87 (group B) pulsatile perfusion was carried out. There were no significant differences between the groups in age, body weight, body surface area, male/female ratio and clinical symptoms (Table 1).

Regarding preoperative cardiac risks, myocardial infarction, previous cardiac operation, ventricular arrhythmias and unstable angina were the main problems in the patients in this study. The preoperative cardiac function was impaired moderately to severely in both groups. There was no significant difference in general operative risk factors between groups except for a higher incidence of carotid artery stenosis and obesity in group B than in group A. The majority of patients (83% in group A; 81% in group B) had more than one risk factor according to Montreal Heart Institution Classification, and they were increased- or high-risk patients.

In group A 13.6% had an isolated cardiac procedure – coronary artery bypass grafting (CABG) or single valve replacement (VR) – and 86.4% had combined procedures like multiple valve replacement, CABG and VR, CABG and thrombendarterectomy (TEA) of internal carotid artery. In group B 17.5% had an isolated cardiac procedure and 82.5% had combined procedures. In 33% of patients from group B carotid TEA was performed combined with CABG and/or VR simultaneously (Table 2).

Regarding perfusion time, ischemic time, total operation time and myocardial protection, there was no significant difference between the groups. In all patients a prolonged period of extracorporeal circulation (longer than 120 min) was necessary, mainly due to combined procedures (Table 3).

Before surgery patients were premedicated with 2 mg noctamid p.o. and 1.5 mg/kg b.w. morphine i.m. Anesthesia was induced with etomidate (0.3–0.5 mg/kg

Table 1. Patient characteristics

Characteristics	NP (*n* = 88)	PP (*n* = 87)
Age (yr)	63.6 ± 8.5	64.6 ± 9.4
Body weight (kg)	68.6 ± 11.6	70.9 ± 9.7
Body surface (m^2)	1.79 ± 0.19	1.82 ± 0.16
Sex (male/female)	74.3%	73.8%
Symptoms (NYHA III/IV)	85.2%	85.7%

Table 2. Operative procedures

Procedures	NP (*n* = 88)	PP (*n* = 87)
Isolated CABG	7.9%	11.1%
Isolated VR	5.7%	6.4%
Multiple VR	11.4%	9.5%
CABG + VR	57.9%	39.7%
CABG + ICA – TEA	17.1%	25.4%
CABG + ICA – TEA + VR	0.0%	7.9%

Table 3. Demographic data

Data	NP (*n* = 88)	PP (*n* = 87)
Perfusion time (min)	151 ± 29	150 ± 27
Ischemic time (min)	77 ± 47	85 ± 35
Operation time (min)	264 ± 74	268 ± 52
Myoc. protection		
Cardioplegia	78.41%	76.19%
Hypothermia	21.59%	23.81%

i.v.) and fentanyl (0.006–0.009 mg/kg i.v.) and vecuronium (0.1 mg/kg i.v.) was used to provide muscle relaxation. After incubation 50% nitrous oxide in oxygen with up to 2 vol% enflurane was used for anesthesia and ventilation. The enflurane given during CPB ranged from 0.6 to 0.8 vol%. In group A standard nonpulsatile perfusion by means of a Stöckert-Shiley roller pump was carried out. In group B a double pump system equipped with a pulsatile flow controller was used for pulsatile perfusion. The pulsatile perfusion was started about 5 min after initiation of CPB. It was continued to the end of the operative procedures and until normothermia was reestablished.

Figure 1 demonstrates our set-up for pulsatile extracorporeal circulation. In order to minimize the hemolytic effects a double pump system was developed and applied. In this system the first pump was inserted between venous drainage

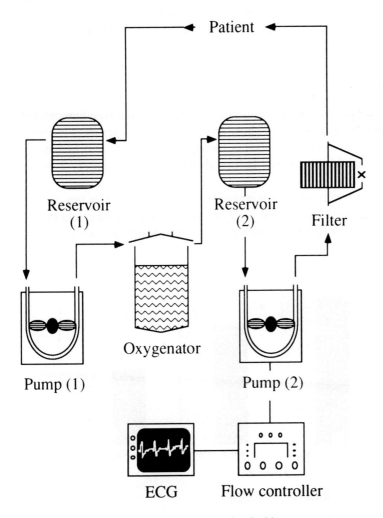

Fig. 1. Set-up for pulsatile perfusion using the double pump system.

and the membrane oxygenator (TMO- HP, Travenol, USA, or MAXIMA, Medtronic, USA) and the second between the oxygenator and the arterial canule in the ascending aorta. The first pump is nonpulsatile and the second is pulsatile. The first pump supplied blood from the venous reservoir through the oxygenator into the arterial reservoir. The second one transported the blood from the arterial reservoir to the aorta. This configuration provides a low mean blood pressure and nonpulsatile flow in the oxygenator so that the sheer forces acting on the erythrocytes in the oxygenator are lower than those present in the conventional single pump devices. For obtaining an early physiological pressure pattern during pulsatile perfusion the diameter of the arterial cannula was chosen with respect to the amount of calculated cardiac output (perfusion rate), namely 8.5 mm in diameter with more than 4.5 l/min cardiac output and 7.5 mm under 4.5 l/min.

During the ECC and the early postoperative period hemolytic factors such as plasma free hemoglobin, hemoglobin, hematocrit, mean arterial pressure, total peripheral vascular resistance, intraoperative net fluid balance and diuresis were estimated. Furthermore, perioperative morbidity and mortality were observed.

Results

The determination of postoperative hemolytic factors – plasma free hemoglobin – 2, 4 and 24 h after surgery did not show any significant differences between the two groups (Fig. 2). Regarding plasma hemoglobin content and hematocrit there was no difference in the periods before, during and after surgery between the two groups.

At 30, 70 and 120 min after beginning ECC the average mean arterial pressures were 66, 72 and 70 mmHg in group A, significantly higher than the 58, 54 and 52 mmHg in group B. The average of mean peripheral vascular resistance

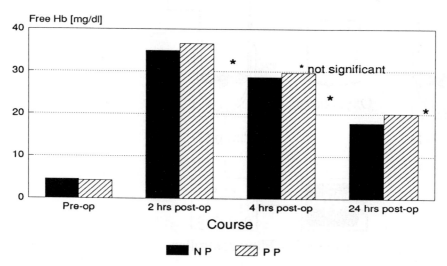

Fig. 2. Plasma free hemoglobin after nonpulsatile (NP) and pulsatile perfusion (PP).

(PVR) determined 5 and 60 min after beginning ECC and 5 min before the end of ECC can be seen in Fig. 3; 60 min after beginning ECC and 5 min before end of ECC the values were significantly higher in group A than in group B (885 vs. 750 dyn·cm^{-5}·s at 60 min, 970 vs. 670 dyn·cm^{-5}·s).

Figure 4 shows a volume/temperature-time diagram in the patients during operation with NP and PP. While with increasing ECC time core temperature (rectal) decreased only slightly, the intraoperative net fluid balance became significantly greater in patients with NP than in patients with PP. At 165, 185 and 195 min of ECC the balance was significantly higher, with 3450, 3750 and 4100 ml in group A compared to 2600, 2700 and 2850 ml in group B, respectively.

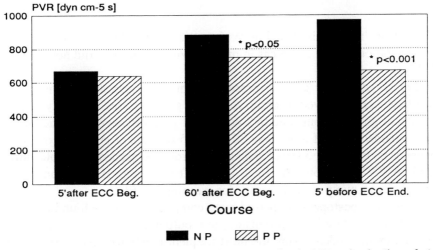

Fig. 3. Peripheral vascular resistance (PVR) during nonpulsatile (NP) and pulsatile perfusion (PP).

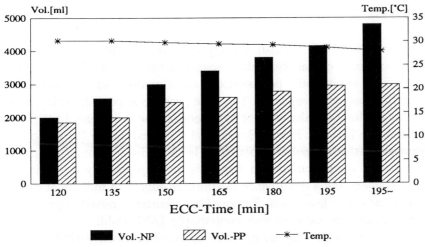

Fig. 4. Volume/temperature-time diagram in the patients during operation with nonpulsatile (NP) and pulsatile perfusion (PP). Vol.-NP, volume supply during NP; Vol.-PP, volume supply during PP; Temp., temperature (nasopharyngeal).

Table 4. Complications

Complications	NP (*n* = 88)	PP (*n* = 87)
Hypertension	14 (16%)	6 (6.8%)
Low output syndrome	8 (9.1%)	0 (0.0%)
Inotropic drugs	31 (35%)	19 (22%)
Renal insufficiency	5 (5.7%)	1 (1.1%)
Cardiac resuscitation	3 (3.5%)	0 (0.0%)
Neurol. deficits	1 (1.1%)	2 (2.3%)
Exitus	2 (2.3%)	2 (2.3%)

One of the main reasons is that diuresis in patients with PP increased proportionally to duration of ECC, whereas in patients with NP diuresis did not increase remarkably.

Immediately after the cardiac procedure (in the operating room) more complications were observed in group A than in group B: low output syndrome in 6 patients of group A compared to 2 patients of group B; severe cardiac failure requiring extended ECC of more than 30 min in 5 patients of group A compared to 2 patients in group B; 38% of patients in group A needed inotropic drugs compared to 23% in group A. In 1 patient from group B insertion of an intraaortic balloon pump was necessary for weaning off ECC.

During the early postoperative period more complications were found in group A than in group B. Arterial hypertension, low output syndrome, renal insufficiency and pulmonary edema were the most frequent complications; 2 patients in each group died due to profound cardiogenic shock (Table 4).

Discussion

The experience with ECC in heart surgery obtained so far indicates that in complex and extensive operations with prolonged perfusion time the use of ECC with conventional nonpulsatile perfusion can occasionally lead to considerable problems in the postoperative period. The main problem is poor diuresis, edema of organs like the lung and the brain or hypertension due to increased peripheral vascular resistance [11–14]. Barratt-Boyes et al. [15] and Sasaki [6] and others could demonstrate that nonpulsatile perfusion leads to disturbance of peripheral organ micro- and lymph circulation which is accompanied by a significant temperature gradient and a disturbance in substrate supply to individual organs resulting in poor organ protection. Tarnow [16] reported a raised migration of fluid in the intestine of patients with nonpulsatile ECC. Boldt et al. [13] and others observed increased lung edema after myocardial revascularization with nonpulsatile ECC leading to a negative postoperative course with prolonged ventilation time. Taylor et al. [11], Landymore et al. [8], Philbin et al. [18] and

Levine et al. [10] reported increased peripheral vascular resistance after NP due to increased activation of angiotensin II or vasopressin, respectively.

In our earlier clinical and experimental studies [7,14] we could demonstrate that the NP compared to PP leads to significantly increased release of endogenic catecholamines by stimulation of sympathetic nerve through carotid baroreceptors and to elevated peripheral vascular resistance. Furthermore, the tendency to edema could be explained by the hypothesis that the increased catecholamine release with NP causes vasoconstriction in the venous capacitive system and thus an increase in mean capillary pressure which leads to a raised filtration pressure and to edema formation.

In our opinion all our data can be explained when the constrictive effects of increased sympathetic tone on the venous system are considered in the light of the fact that the vessel wall muscularization and the number of adrenergic receptors in the vessel walls increase along the course of the veins. The larger venules (venules of second and first order) in the capacitive system with more pronounced musculature and higher amount of adrenergic receptors manifest a

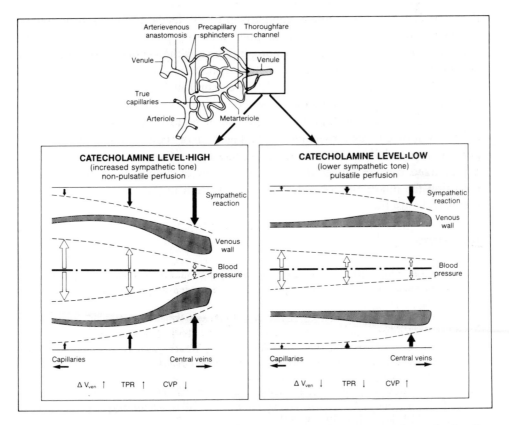

Fig. 5. Proposed mechanism of the response of the venous capacitive system to adrenergic stimuli. ΔV_{ven}, change of venous blood volume; TPR, total peripheral resistence; CVP, central venous volume.

74

more pronounced response to the effect of sympathetic tone [18-20]. As Fig. 5 shows, the constriction of these vessels has a 'throttle effect' with respect to the blood flow in small postcapillary venules (mainly nonmuscular – 'third order' venules) and causes an increased pressure in this section of circulation. The raised venous pressure counteracts not only the contractile effect of the sympathetic tone but finally leads to an observed volume increase in the capacitive system as well as to raised capillary pressure and thus to a rise in filtration pressure which in turn results in increased tendency to edema formation.

As demonstrated on the right-hand side of Fig. 5, a lower sympathetic tone with PP eliminates the 'throttle effect' in the larger venules. This on the one hand results in a tendency to increase in central venous pressure, and on the other hand leads to a pressure reduction in the small postcapillary venules and thus to a volume reduction in the capacitive system, a lowered filtration pressure in capillaries and finally to a reduced tendency to edema formation.

Summary

It can be concluded that NP, in comparison to PP, leads to increased peripheral vascular resistance, which leads to poor diuresis, poor microcirculation and disturbed cardiac function. Furthermore, it increases the venous capacitive system as well with marked loss of intravascular volume and edema formation due to raised filtration pressure. Consequently the cerebral and pulmonary function could be impaired during the perioerative period.

These results suggest that the routine use of pulsatile perfusion during ECC offers significant hemodynamic advantages over conventional nonpulsatile perfusion, especially in patients with increased operative risk and/or undergoing a prolonged cardiac procedure. For elimination of hemolysis during pulsatile perfusion the integration of a double pump system in the extracorporeal circuit seems to be useful.

References

1. Jacobs LA, Klopp EH, Searmore W, Toparz SR, Gott VL (1969) Improved organ function during cardiac bypass with roller pump modified to deliver pulsatile flow. Surgery 58: 703-712.
2. Trinkle JK, Helton NE, Wood RE, Bryant WR (1969) Metabolic comparison of a new pulsatile pump and a roller pump for cardiopulmonary bypass. J Thorac Cardiovasc Surg 58: 562-569.
3. German JC, Chalmers GS, Hirai J, Mukherjee ND, Wakabayashi A, Connolly JE (1972) Comparison of nonpulsatile and pulsatile extracorporal circulation on renal tissue perfusion. Chest 61: 65-69.
4. Arnold G, Kosche F, Miessner E, Neitzert A, Lochner W (1968) The importance of the perfusion pressure in the coronary arteries for the contractility and the oxygen consumption of the heart. Pflügers Arch 299: 339-343.
5. Körfer R, Steven W, Frenzel H, Arnold G, Bircks W (1980) Pulsatile versus nonpulsatile coronary perfusion in the fibrillating canine heart. E.S.A.O. Proc 34-38.

75

6. Sasaki Y (1977) Perfusion cooling by pulsatile flow. Jpn J Surg 7: 960-1004.

7. Minami K, Körner MM, Vyska K, Kleesiek K, Knobl H, Körfer R (1990) Effects of pulsatile perfusion on plasma catecholamine levels and hemodynamics during and after cardiac surgery using cardiopulmonary bypass. J Thorac Cardiovasc Surg 99: 82-91.

8. Landymore RW, Murphy DA, Kinley E (1981) Does pulsatile flow improve glucose tolerance during extracorporeal circulation? J Cardiovasc Surg 22: 239-244.

9. Wada Y, Sasaki Y, Kadowaki M, Kitaura K, Nishiyama K, Hashimoto T, Shirakata S, Oga K, Oka T (1986) Clinical studies on pulsatile perfusion cooling for open heart surgery. Jpn J Thorac Surg 34: 79-83.

10. Levine FH, Philbin DM, Kono K (1981) Plasma vasopressin levels and urinary sodium excretion during cardiopulmonary bypass with and without pulsatile flow. Ann Thorac Surg 32: 63-67.

11. Taylor KM, Bain WH, Russell M, Brannan JJ, Morten JJ (1979) Peripheral vascular resistance and angiotensin II levels during pulsatile and non-pulsatile cardiopulmonary bypass. Thorax 34: 594-598.

12. Duma St, Aksakal D, Benzer W, Haider W, Krieger G, Palzer K, Schuhfried F (1985) Intraoperative Veränderunger des extravaskulären Lungenwassers. Anaesthesist 34: 593-597.

13. Boldt T, v. Bormann B, Kling D, Görlich G, Hempelmann G (1985) Der Einfluss der Beatmung mit unterschiedlich hohem endexspiratorischen Druck auf das extravaskuläre Lungenwasser (EVLW) nach extrakorporaler Zirkulation. Anaesthesist 34: 287-292.

14. Minami K, Thompson T, Notohamiprodjo G, Körner MM, Körfer R (1990) Einfluss der pulsatilen und nichtpulsatilen extrakorporalen Zirkulation auf Flüssigkeitretention nach aortocoronarer Bypassoperation. Z Kardiol 83 (Suppl 1): 131.

15. Barratt-Boyes BG, Simpson M, Neutze JM (1971) Intracardiac surgery in neonates and infants using deep hypothermia with surface cooling and limited cardiopulmonary bypass. Circulation 43 (Suppl I): 25-30.

16. Tarnow T (1983) Anaesthesie und Kardiologie in der Herzchirurgie. Berlin: Springer.

17. Philbin DM, Levine FH, Kong K, et al. (1981) Attenuation of stress response to cardiopulmonary bypass by the addition of pulsatile flow. Circulation 64: 808-812.

18. Faber EJ (1988) In situ analysis of alpha-adrenoceptors on arteriolar and venular smooth muscle in rat skeletal muscle microcirculation. Circ Res 62: 37-50.

19. Martin HW, Tolley KT, Saffitz EJ (1990) Autoradiographic delineation of skeletal muscle alpha-1-adrenergic receptor distribution. Am J Physiol 259: 1402-1408.

20. Renkin EM (1984) Control of microcirculation and blood-tissue exchange. In: Handbook of Physiology, section 2: The Cardiovascular System, Volume IV, part 2. Bethesda, MD: American Physiological Society, 627-687.

Cardio-thoracic surgery. K. Minami et al. editors.

Blood use in cardiac surgery

E. Wolner, J. Schneider and M. Havel
II. Surgical Clinic, University of Vienna, Spitalgasse 23, 1090 Vienna, Austria

Introduction

The increasing need for blood and blood products in cardiac surgery has led to a great strain on the resources of blood banks throughout the world. Although the mean blood use per cardiac operation has significantly declined over the last few years, the increasing number of cardiac operations performed has led to an exponential rise in the need for blood. In 1971 the mean blood requirement per patient was 8 units [1]. Newer studies show that 70% of all cardiac operations can be performed without the use of foreign blood [2]. Nevertheless, today the mean blood use per cardiac operation remains at 2 units [3].

Aside from the strain on finances and personnel, each blood product used carries potential dangers with it. These dangers include small risks of allergic reactions (1:100), the transfer of viral hepatitis (1:200), hemolytic transfusion reactions (1:6000), or the transfer of HIV infection (1:150,000).

Especially in the third world the transfer of malaria through blood products represents a significant problem. More than 15% of all potential blood donors are infected with malaria [4]. The transfer of Chagas disease presents a particular problem in South and Central America. Further infectious problems include syphilis, cytomegalovirus and Epstein Barr virus.

Heart, lung and kidney failure after multiple transfusions is also a recognized problem.

From the above-mentioned problems, it follows that the surest way to reduce the complications associated with foreign blood contact is the avoidance of foreign blood contact. Numerous technical and pharmacologic methods of blood conservation are available.

Blood conservation techniques

Autologous blood donation

A variety of methods exist for the withdrawal and storage of autologous blood preoperatively, intraoperatively and postoperatively. Before routine operations, before the patient is hospitalized, the patient can donate his own blood. Blood may also be taken before the beginning of extracorporeal circulation. Intraoperatively, processing through the Cell-Saver may be used. The reinfusion of blood from postoperative drains is a further possibility.

Preoperative autologous blood donation

For electively planned surgical operations, in the absence of contraindications, the donation of autologous blood is the best method of obtaining blood products. The following factors are considered contraindications; body weight under 50 kg, poor general condition, infectious diseases, epilepsy, anemia (HgB < 12.5 g/100 ml), unstable angina pectoris, aortic stenosis, LVEF < 45%, maximal exercise capacity under 50 W, and rhythm disturbances.

Autologous blood donated before the hospitalization can either be stored at 5°C, after the addition of citrate, or the erythrocytes can be frozen after separation. The total volume which can be donated by a patient depends on the maximal storage time and on the ability to stimulate the erythropoetic system. The intravenous administration of iron or erythropoeitin can significantly increase erythrocyte synthesis.

Another possibility for increasing the yield in autologous blood donation, especially when there are contraindications to erythrocyte freezing, is the 'piggyback technique'. With this method, within 6 weeks 4 units of erythrocyte concentrate and 6 units of fresh frozen plasma (FFP) can be harvested. Six weeks before the planned operation the first unit of blood is taken. This is separated into erythrocytes, which are stored at 5°C, and FFP, which is frozen. Two weeks later, the stored erythrocytes are reinfused and simultaneously two units are withdrawn. This sequence, withdrawal, storage, reinfusion, and subsequent increased withdrawal, is carried out a total of four times [5].

In patients in whom there are no contraindications to blood freezing, the nearly time-unlimited storage of blood products in liquid nitrogen is certainly a good method. However, the resistance to hemolysis of blood cells treated in such a manner is lower [6]. Further, the sensitivity of cells so treated to osmotic swelling is also significantly increased, comparable to that seen in spherocytosis. For this reason, erythrocytes which have been stored in liquid nitrogen should not be used in patients with decreased kidney function [7]. The use of frozen blood products during extracorporeal circulation has not been shown to influence the prothrombin time (PTT), the fibrinogen or thrombocyte function.

Intraoperative autologous blood use

Withdrawal of autologous blood intraoperatively, immediately before the beginning of extracorporeal circulation, is already a widely used method.

The withdrawn blood is reinfused immediately after the end of extracorporeal circulation. Numerous studies have shown that intraoperative autologous blood reinfusion significantly decreases the need for heterologous blood [8]. Hallowell and co-workers showed that the requirement for foreign blood was reduced by 25% with this method [9]. Other studies showed that platelet count and platelet adhesion were better in those patients who had received autologous blood [10].

Wagstaffe and co-workers showed that anticoagulation with acid-citrate-dextrose (ACD) was superior to anticoagulation with heparin [11]. Patients who received ACD-treated autologous blood had significantly higher platelet counts and less bleeding postoperatively.

Other investigators demonstrated that blood removal from the V. cava was superior to that using the A. radialis or the V. jugularis [4]. Despite these controversial experimental results, the withdrawal of autologous blood from the venous line of the heart-lung machine immediately after the beginning of cardiopulmonary bypass is certainly the method most widely used due to the ease of its performance. The autologous blood is stored at room temperature in the operation room until its reinfusion.

The following formula is used to calculate the blood volume which may be withdrawn:

$$DV = ((0.07 \ BW \times (Hct \ pt - Hct \ bp) - (Hct \ bp \times OV))/Hct \ pt$$

DV = donated volume, BW = body weight, Hct pt = patient hemotocrit, Hct bp = hematocrit during bypass, and OV = oxygenator volume.

Intraoperative autologous blood donation appears justified only in patients with a hematocrit of over 30% and a withdrawal volume of 500 ml, supporting a hematocrit of 25% during extracorporeal circulation.

Reinfusion of oxygenator blood
The reinfusion of oxygenator blood is a recognized routine procedure in cardiac surgery. In numerous patients, however, it is impossible to reinfuse the entire volume without the risk of hypervolemia. Studies comparing oxygenator blood to 14-day-old blood products demonstrated that oxygenator blood was superior with respect to pH, potassium and calcium concentrations, as well as having a lower plasma hemoglobin level [13]. The hematocrit of oxygenator blood was, however, significantly lower. Therefore the principal disadvantages of oxygenator blood lie in the lower hematocrit and the higher heparin content. These disadvantages can be overcome by centrifuging the oxygenator blood.

Autotransfusion systems
Intraoperative After protamine is given, further suctioning of blood into the heart-lung machine must be discontinued to avoid blood coagultion in the heart-lung machine. Parker described a system in which a connection between the cardiotomy reservoir and the arterial line proximal to the oxygenator was made [14]. This system found earlier use in operations such as acute aortic dissection or reoperations in which a greater blood loss is expected. With this and similar systems local anticoagulation must be added.

Blood which is suctioned directly from the operative field has a low hematocrit, high free hemoglobin, high concentration of oxygen radicals, and high concentration of LDH, GOT, creatine kinase and bilirubin. However, the advantage of a high platelet concentration remains.

Cell-Saver With the introduction of the Cell-Saver, and with it the possibility of immediate centrifugation and washing of blood suctioned from the surgical field, numerous disadvantages of older autotransfusion systems were overcome. Through the washing and centrifugation process, injured platelets, leukocytes, free hemoglobin and heparin are removed. Simultaneously the hematocrit rises due to the concentration effect.

Postoperative reinfusion of drainage blood The postoperative reinfusion of mediastinal drainage was studied in detail at the Johns Hopkins Hospital [15,16]. The investigators found an extremely cost-effective system which was free of major complications. By reinfusing mediastinal blood the requirement for heterologous blood transfusion decreased from 8.4 to 4.2 units. It could be shown that the filter used had no effect on the hematocrit, but did lead to a decrease in platelets and leukocytes. In comparison to heterologous blood products, the reinfused mediastinal blood had a lower hematocrit, a higher platelet concentration, lower fibrinogen, and a higher concentration of fibrin split products. However, the concentrations of Factor VII and IX were higher. Despite the lower fibrinogen concentrations and the presence of fibrin split products, no evidence of consumption coagulopathy was found.

Hemodilution

Hemodilution is today an established component of the technique of extracorporeal circulation. In addition to the blood-sparing aspects, hemodilution has a positive influence on the postoperative lung and kidney function, on blood coagulation, and on myocardial function [15]. Normally, hematocrits of 20–30% are achieved. However, more extreme values of 11–18% may be reached without injury to the patient. The occurrence of positive postoperative fluid balance can be decreased by the use of albumin. The safe degree of hemodilution also depends substantially on the temperature of the perfusate, i.e. the lower the temperature, the lower the acceptable hematocrit.

An important factor for the execution of hemodilution is the patient's blood volume. Significant differences are found between the individual cardiac diseases. The blood volume is higher in patients with an LVEF < 40%. Patients with valve disease have a higher blood volume in comparison to patients with coronary disease. Similarly, the blood volume increases with the number of diseased valves.

Pharmacologic methods

Aprotinin
Aprotinin is an inhibitor of human trypsin, plasmin, and kallikrein. In 1987 Royston et al. proved that aprotinin (280 mg added to the heart-lung machine, 280 mg as a loading dose after the beginning of anaesthesia, and 70 mg/h as a

continuous infusion until the end of the operation) significantly decreased both the postoperative bleeding and blood transfusion requirements in cardiac reoperations [17]. These results were confirmed by others. In particular, Bidstrup et al. advocated the use of the high-dose aprotinin method [18]. In our own investigations on patients undergoing primary orthotopic heart transplantation we showed that a lower dose of aprotinin (560 mg) also resulted in a significant reduction in postoperative bleeding. Seventy percent of the transplantations in the aprotinin group could be carried out without heterologous transfusion. This was possible in only 30% in the control group. Correspondingly, the amount of postoperative bleeding in the aprotinin group was significantly less (510 ml vs. 820 ml, $p < 0.01$; 690 ml vs. 1000 ml, $p < 0.03$; 24 and 48 h postoperatively respectively) [19].

We performed a further double-blind study in 120 patients. It could again be shown that a lower dose of aprotinin had a comparable blood-sparing effect. In this study 40 patients received 6.0×10^6 KIU aprotinin (2.0×10^6 KIU as an initial bolus followed by 2.0×10^6 KIU as a continuous infusion and 2.0×10^6 KIU in the heart-lung machine), 40 patients received only 2×10^6 KIU aprotinin in the heart-lung machine, and 40 patients received a placebo. The patients in the aprotinin group demonstrated a significantly lower bleeding tendency and a correspondingly lower transfusion requirement than the placebo group. No difference could be found between the two aprotinin groups.

The exact mechanism of action of aprotinin has only been partially clarified. Van Oeveren et al. reported a protection of platelet factor glycoprotein Ib by aprotinin during the initial phase of extracorporeal circulation [20].

Our studies indicated that aprotinin inhibited fibrinolysis [21]. In studies on human endothelial cells which had been incubated with different concentrations of aprotinin, it could be proven that aprotinin inhibited the release of 6-keto-prostaglandin $F_{1\alpha}$ and simultaneously increased the synthesis and release of thromboxane B_2 and von Willebrand factor [22,23].

These results, and the theoretical extensions thereof, led to the conclusion that the use of aprotinin during aortocoronary bypass operations could lead to a reduction in the rate of bypass occlusion. Based on this, we undertook a randomized, double-blind study of 45 patients undergoing complex aortocoronary bypass operations. Fifteen patients received no aprotinin, 15 patients received 2.0×10^6 KIU aprotinin, and 15 patients received 6.0×10^6 KIU aprotinin. All patients were reangiogrammed between 8 and 10 dyas postoperatively. There were no differences seen in the bypass occlusion rate between the three groups.

Epoprostenol (Prostaclycin PGI₂)

PGI₂ stimulates platelet adenylate cyclase, increases the platelet cAMP concentration, and inhibits platelet aggregation. Paradoxically, it can reduce the blood loss after cardiac operations. During cardiopulmonary bypass (CPB) the platelet count declines, in part due to hemodilution, but also as a consequence of aggregation due to contact with the nonbiologic surface and through sequestration in the liver or spleen. The administration of epoprostenol at the time of heparinization before the beginning of CPB leads to an increase in platelet count during extracorporeal circulation and also on the first postoperative day. The bleeding time 1 h after the end of the operation is significantly reduced. Nevertheless, the clinical benefit in terms of a decrease in postoperative blood loss has been disappointing.

Desmopressin

Desmopressin increases the plasma concentration and the activity of the high molecular forms of Factor VIII, of von Willebrand Factor, which is necessary for the adhesion of platelets to the subintimal connective tissue and which shortens the bleeding time of patients with Willebrand-Juerges syndrome with thrombopathy. However, the bleeding time and the partial thromboplastin time are also shortened in normal humans. Factor VIII can be adsorbed onto nonbiologic surfaces. By this method an enhancement in coagulation after CPB can be expected. Patients receiving desmopressin demonstrated a mean decrease in blood product use of 30% compared to patients receiving placebo. The platelet count was also significantly higher postoperatively in the desmopressin group.

Diverse methods

Fibrin glue

Fibrin glue was used for the first time world-wide at the University of Vienna II Surgical Clinic in 1976. This two-component glue can either be sprayed as a thin film over a large diffusely bleeding area or can be applied with a collagen sponge for control of circumscribed sources of bleeding which are not surgically manageable.

Especially important is the use of fibrin glue to seal non-precoated vessel prostheses such as those used in operations for thoracic aneurysms.

Final comments

By combining different blood-sparing methods it is possible today to perform almost all routine open-heart operations without the use of heterologous blood. However, only a few centers are able to use all the state-of-the-art techniques for blood conservation. Therefore, appropriate methods must be chosen according to the requirements and experience of the individual institutions.

References

1. Roche JK, Stengle JM (1973) J Am Med Assoc 225: 1516.
2. Zubiate P, Kay JH, Mendez AM (1974) J Thorac Cardiovasc Surg 68: 263.
3. Cosgrove DM, Thurer RL, Lytle BW (1979) Ann Thorac Surg 28: 184.
4. Cohen ND, Munoz A, Reitz B (1989) N Engl J Med 320: 1172.

5. Utley JR, Moores WY, Stephens DB (1981) Ann Thorac Surg 31: 482.
6. Valeri CR, Bougas JA, Talarico L (1970) Transfusion 10: 238.
7. Hanson EL, Fosberg AM (1972) J Thorac Cardiovasc Surg 64: 87.
8. Hallowell P, Bland JHL, Dalton BC (1978) Ann Thorac Surg 25: 22.
9. Hallowell P, Bland JHL, Chir B (1972) J Thorac Cardiovasc Surg 64: 941.
10. Hardesty RL, Bayer WL, Bahnson HT (1968) J Thorac Cardiovasc Surg 56: 683.
11. Wagstaffe JG, Clarke AD (1972) Thorax 27: 410.
12. Kaplan JA, Cannarella C, Jones EL (1977) J Thorac Cardiovasc Surg 74: 4.
13. Tarhan S, Moffitt EA, Lundborg RO (1970) Surgery 67: 584.
14. Parker FB, West H (1978) Ann Thorac Surg 26: 559.
15. Roe BB, Swenson EE, Hepps SA (1964) Arch Surg 88: 128.
16. Schaff HV, Hauer JM, Bell WR (1978) J Thorac Cardiovasc Surg 75: 632.
17. Royston D, Bidstrup BP, Taylor KM (1987) Lancet 1290.
18. Bidstrup BP, Royston D, Sapsford RN (1989) J Thorac Cardiovasc Surg 97: 364.
19. Havel M, Owen A, Simon P (in press) J Heart Lung Transplant.
20. van Oeveren W, Harder MP (1990) J Thorac Cardiovasc Surg 99: 788.
21. Havel M, Teufelsbauer H, Knoebl P (1991) J Thorac Cardiovasc Surg 101: 968.
22. Havel M, Griesmacher A, Weigel G (in press) J Thorac Cardiovasc Surg.
23. Havel M, Griesmacher A, Weigel G (in press) Surgery.

Reduction of blood use in 'redos' of coronary artery bypass grafting: double-blind study with administration of aprotinin

K. Minami, H. Buschler, M. Hoffmann, G. Notohamiprodjo, G. Mayer and R. Körfer

Department of Thoracic and Cardiovascular Surgery, Heart Center North Rhine–Westphalia, University of Bochum, 4970 Bad Oeynhausen, Georgstrasse 11, F.R.G.

Introduction

The risk of transmission of infection with several pathogenic organisms is one of the troublesome complications after transfusion of donor blood [1]. Demand for blood transfusion increases depending on age of the patients, preoperative clinical state, duration of extracorporeal circulation performed and type of operative procedure. The increasing number of elderly patients causes more complicated operations such as combined and/or redo procedures. Therefore a growing interest in methods to reduce the need for blood transfusions in cardiac surgery is obvious [2].

Early clinical trials to reduce blood transfusion concentrated on mechanical questions. Besides improvement of operative techniques isovolemic hemodilution with autotransfusion, use of cell saver, cell separator and retransfusion of shed mediastinal blood were recommended [3]. In our clinic only hemodilution with retransfusion of oxygenator blood is used. But investigations have now shifted to pharmacological methods like administration of prostacyclin, desmopresin acetate, epsilon aminocaproic acid and recently low- and high-dose aprotinin [4–7].

It was one aim of our double-blind study to evaluate whether it would be possible to achieve additional reduction of blood loss by administration of aprotinin (Trasylol®, Bayer AG, Leverkusen). We selected patients undergoing repeat (redo) myocardial revascularization, since these patients are usually candidates for donor blood transfusion. Another aim was to obtain further information about the mechanisms of action of this agent.

Patients and Methods

In 54 patients scheduled for elective repeat myocardial revascularization a double-blind study was performed. Aprotinin and placebo were provided by the manufacturer (Bayer AG, Leverkusen, Germany) in identical packages, each containing 12 bottles marked with random numbers. Each bottle of aprotinin contained 500,000 kallikrein inactivator units (KIU) (= 70 mg) aprotinin in 50 ml 0.9% saline solution, and the placebo bottles contained only saline. After introduction of anaesthesia and beginning of skin incision the patients received a loading dose of 2×10^6 KIU aprotinin over a 15 min period followed by a continuous infusion of 500,000 KIU aprotinin per hour during and up to the end of operation. An additional bolus dose of 2×10^6 KIU aprotinin was added to the priming volume of the membrane oxygenator (Maxima®, Medtronic, Minneapolis, USA) in the heart-lung machine. Patients in the control group received the same volume of saline solution.

Before surgery patients were premedicated with 2 mg noctamid p.o. and 1.5 mg/kg b.w. morphine i.m. Anaesthesia was induced with etomidate (0.3–0.5 mg/kg i.v.) and fentanyl (0.006–0.009 mg/kg i.v.) and vecuronium (0.1 mg/kg i.v.) was used to provide muscle relaxation. After intubation 50% nitrous oxide in oxygen with up to 1.5 vol% enflurane was used for anaesthesia and ventilation. The enflurane given during CPB ranged from 0.6 to 0.8 vol%.

A dose of 500 U/kg of mucosa heparin (Braun Melsungen AG, Melsungen, FRG) was injected via a central venous catheter before cannulation of aorta and right atrium. Further heparin (100–125 U/kg) was administered when the activated clotting time (ACT) decreased under 400 s. In all patients the extracorporeal system consisted of a membrane oxygenator (Maxima®, Medtronic, St. Paul, USA) and a roller pump (Stöckert-Shiley®, Munich, FRG) primed with a 2000 ml Ringer-Lactate solution. After beginning of ECC colloidal solution (Osmofundin® 20%, B. Braun Melsungen AG, FRG; 2.3 ml × body weight [kg]) was substituted additionally. Cardiopulmonary bypass (CPB) was performed at a rate of 2.4 $l/min/ml^{-2}$. For myocardial protection moderate systemic hypothermia (blood temperature 27°C) was performed with intermittent cross-clamping of the aorta. The necessary volume for CPB was added to the circulating volume initially by infusion of Ringer-Lactate solution and later by transfusion of donor blood to maintain the hematocrit over 28% and the hemoglobin content over 9.0 g/dl. After completion of CPB residual heparin was neutralized with protamine chloride initially at a ratio of 1.0 to the dose of heparin and additionally 100–125 U/kg protamine to obtain the ACT in normal range (120–140 s). Residual blood in the extracorporeal circuit was collected in the bag containing citric acid and all of the collected packed blood was transfused back to the patients as a blood and/or volume replacement up to 4 h after surgery.

All except 3 patients in this study were operated upon by one surgeon with the same operating team, and bleeding tendency at the time of chest closure was judged by the same team.

Intraoperative blood loss was assessed by measuring the content of the suction reservoir and weighing the gauzes. Postoperative blood loss via the chest tubes was measured 6, 12 and 24 h after surgery. The indication for transfusion during the intra- and postoperative period was defined as a hemoglobin content under 9.0 g/% or a hemtocrit less than 28%.

To determine the mechanism of action of aprotinin several hematological parameters such as activated clotting time (ACT), prothrombin time (PTT), thrombin time (TT), activated partial prothrombin time (aPTT), antithrombin III and alpha-2 plasmin inhibitor-plasmin complex (alpha-2 PI-Pm C). For the quantitation of alpha-2 PI-Pm C, which is an indicator of activation of plasmin-induced fibrinolytic process [8,9], the PIC-test (Teijin Institute, Tokyo, Japan) developed by Aoki et al. (1987) was used [10,11]. This is an enzyme immune assay using monoclonal antibodies against alpha-2 plasmin inhibitor [12–14].

Blood samples were collected from the central venous catheter or the arterial end of the oxygenator at the following times: (1) before anaesthesia, (2) 5 min after surgical incision before administration of heparin, (3) 5 min and (4) 30 min after beginning CPB, (5) shortly before ending CPB, (6) 2 h, (7) 4 h and (8) 24 h after surgery.

Student's t test was used for statistical analysis of demographic data, blood loss and hematologic examinations and Fisher's exact test was performed for analysis of the need of transfusion and perioperative complications.

Results

Two patients in the aprotinin group and 3 patients in the placebo group were eliminated from the statistical evaluation of this study due to the following reasons: intraoperative bleeding from right ventricle at thoracotomy and postoperative bleeding due to displacement of hemoclip on IMA graft; resuscitation at thoracotomy; pleural blood loss which was recognized after administration of protamin; one patient in placebo group received aprotinin inadvertently in postoperative period (Table 1).

Table 2 shows demographic data of the patients who were accepted for statistical evaluation. Regarding age, body weight, height, operation time and ECC time, there was no significant difference between groups.

Cumulative thoracic drainage volume can be seen in Fig. 1. Total blood loss was 132, 191, 313 ml at 6, 12, 24 h after surgery in aprotinin group and 323, 424 and 590 ml in placebo group, respectively. The blood loss was significantly lower in patients with aprotinin than in patients from placebo group ($p < 0.01$) during

Table 1. Drop out patients

Causes	Aprotinin group ($n = 2/28$)	Placebo group ($n = 3/26$)
Surgical bleeding		
Rupture of RV	1	0
Displacement of clip	0	1
Pleural blood loss	0	1
Resuscitation	1	0
Administr. of hemostatic drug	0	1

RV, right ventricle.

88

the total perioperative period.

Figure 2 demonstrates the percentage of patients who received a blood transfusion. In 72% of patients from aprotinin group transfusion of donor blood was not necessary, whereas it was in 48% in placebo group; 7% of patients from aprotinin group needed blood transfusion of 1–3 units and 2% more than 3 units, compared to 31% and 8%, respectively, in placebo group.

Figure 3 shows maximum, minimum and average hematocrit of both groups at 3 different stages in the postoperative period. Average of the mean hematocrit in each group was over 30% at all stages. At no stage did the minimum hematocrit in aprotinin group drop below the critical level of 28%.

Table 2. Demographic data of patients

Data	Aprotinin group (n = 26)	Placebo group (n = 23)
Age (yr)	59.0 ± 8.6	60.6 ± 7.6
Body weight (kg)	75.6 ± 11.2	77.7 ± 10.8
Body height (cm)	174.4 ± 8.1	172.7 ± 6.7
Operation time (min)	228.4 ± 39.3	221.6 ± 38.5
ECC time (min)	86.9 ± 34.6	76.1 ± 24.1

ECC, Extracorporeal circulation.

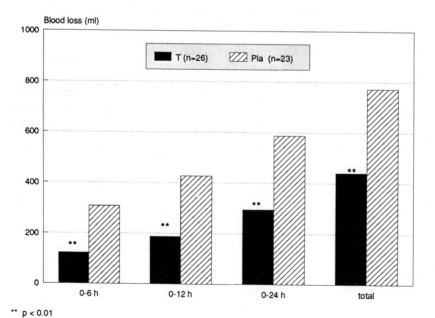

** p < 0.01

Fig. 1. Cumulative thoracic drainage after surgery: The blood loss was significantly lower in patients with aprotinin than in patients from placebo group (*p* < 0.01) during the total perioperative period.

Perioperative complications in both groups can be seen in Table 3. Three patients in aprotinin group suffered from myocardial infarction including one patient with markedly calcified ascending aorta. No patient in placebo group had myocardial infarction perioperatively. There was no other serious complications in both groups.

The plasma levels of aprotinin concentration rose to a mean value of 275 KIU, ranging from 230 to 350 KIU 5 min after beginning ECC, and decreased to 154 KIU, ranging from 120 to 200 KIU at the end of ECC. Figure 4 shows the relationship between blood loss and plasma levels of aprotinin 5 min after beginning ECC. These data indicate that there is an inverse correlation between these two parameters; i.e., the blood loss was significantly lower at higher plasma levels of aprotinin.

Alpha-2 PI-Pm complex was significantly higher in placebo group than in

Table 3. Complications

Complications	Aprotinin group (n = 26)	Placebo group (n = 23)
Pulmonary insufficiency	1	1
Myocardial infarction	3*	0
Renal insufficiency	0	1
Inotropic drugs	1	2
Allergic reaction	0	0

*One of these had markedly calcified ascending aorta.

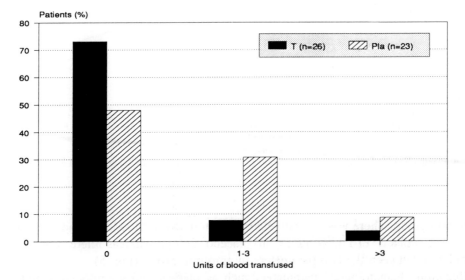

Fig. 2. Donor blood transfusion. In 72% of patients from aprotinin group transfusion of donor blood was not necessary, whereas it was in in 48% in placebo group.

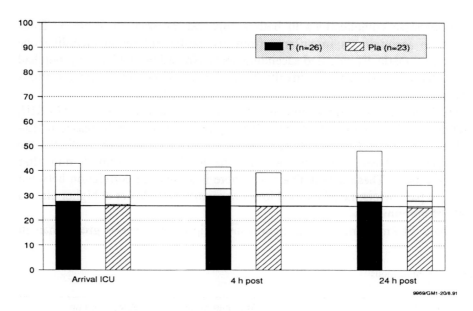

Fig. 3. Hematocrit of both groups at 3 different stages in the postoperative period.

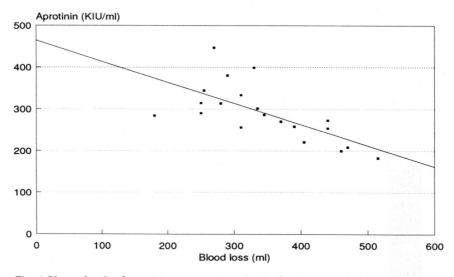

Fig. 4. Plasma levels of aprotinin concentration (5 min after beginning ECC) and blood loss in the aprotinin group.

aprotinin group. There was a positive correlation between blood loss and plasma levels of alpha-2 PI-Pm complex in placebo group, whereas there was no correlation between the two parameters in aprotinin group (Fig. 5).

Regarding hematological parameters such as platelet and granulocyte count, hematocrit, hemoglobin content, pGOT, pGPT, total protein, urea and creatinin,

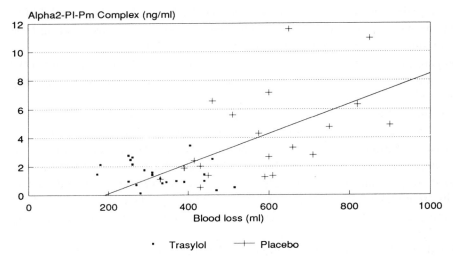

Fig. 5. Alpha-2 PI-Pm complex in aprotinin and placebo group.

there was no difference between groups. There was enhanced prolongation of activated clotting time in aprotinin group.

Discussion

Causes of increased bleeding after cardiac surgery using CPB are numerous and varied, and difficult to characterize. The complexity of this problem is related to the hemostatic process, effects of pharmacological agents, operative procedure and technique, hypothermia, hemodilution, and type of oxygenator. It is well known that fibrin formation – coagulation – and fibrinolysis occur simultaneously during hemostasis, but imbalance between these two different forces influences the occurrence of thrombogenic disorders and bleeding.

The results of our clinical study in patients undergoing repeat myocardial revascularization have shown that the average blood loss in patients treated with aprotinin was nearly half of that lost in patients from placebo group. Consequently, need for donor blood transfusion after surgery until discharge of patients was markedly reduced in patients with aprotinin; 72% of patients in aprotinin group received no transfusion compared to 48% of patients in placebo group. The plasma aprotinin concentration, which had been raised to over 250 KIU 5 min after beginning CPB and kept in the range between 120 and 200 KIU up to end of the CPB, demonstrated that there was an inverse correlation between blood loss and aprotinin concentration.

Regarding the mechanism of action of aprotinin several explanations are found in the literature. Provoc-Cernic suggested marked inhibition of proteolysis and fibrinolysis, having found increased fibrin degradation products. Fritz, Royston, Fraedrich and Bidstrup proposed direct or indirect prevention of platelet function or aggregation. In a recently published study Dietrich et al. focussed on inhibition of the contact phase of coagulation indicating prolonged activated clotting time (ACT) and activated partial thromboplastin time (aPTT).

Regarding cardiac complications, there was an increased rate of perioperative infarction, namely 3 patients with perioperative infarction in the aprotinin group compared to no infarction in the placebo group.

The alpha-2 PI-Pm complex was significantly increased in the placebo group. There was a positive relationship between blood loss and plasma concentration of alpha-2 PI-Pm complex. These findings showed that the increased alpha-2 PI-Pm complex is accompanied by a bleeding tendency due to activated fibrinolysis. Seitz et al. [27] and Aoki et al. [10] suggested in their experimental and clinical studies that alpha-2 PI-Pm complex is the major end-product of activation of the plasminogen system and the increased levels indicate a state of ongoing fibrinolysis.

Whatever the mechanism of action, administration of this agent, which leads to decreased blood loss and thereby decreased need for donor blood transfusion, seems to be useful especially in patients undergoing prolonged extracorporeal circulation. But how much the decreased level of fibrinolytic activity with administration of aprotinin has an influence on thrombogenic complications in bypass grafts could be answered in a larger series of patients treated with this agent.

References

1. Colloins JD, Bassendine MF, Codd AA, Collins A, Ferner RE, James OF (1983) Prospective study of posttransfusion hepatitis after cardiac surgery in a British centre. Br Med J 287: 1422–1424.
2. Woodman RC, Harker LA (1990) Bleeding complications associated with cardiopulmonary bypass. Blood 9: 1680–1697.
3. Schlosser V, Kuttler H, Johannesson T, Schindler M (1987) Herz- und gefässchirurgische Eingriffe ohne Fremdbluttransfusionen. Herz/Kreislauf 19: 400–403.
4. Alajmo F, Calamai G, Perna AM, et al. (1989) High-dose aprotinin: hemostatic effects in open heart operations. Ann Thorac Surg 48: 536–539.
5. Covino E, Pepino P, Marino L, Ferrara P, Spampinato N (1991) Low dose aprotinin as blood saver in open heart surgery. Eur J Cardio-thorac Surg 5: 414–418.
6. Dietrich W, Barankay A, Dilthey G, Henze R, Niekau E, et al. (1989) Reduction of homologous blood requirement in cardiac surgery by intraoperative aprotinin application-clinical experience in 152 cardiac surgical patients. Thorac Cardiovasc Surg 37: 92–98.
7. Fish KJ, Sarnquist FH, Steennis C van, Mitchell RS, Hilberman M, et al. (1986) A prospective, randomized study of the effects of prostacyclin on platelets and blood loss during coronary bypass operations. J Thorac Cardiovasc Surg 91: 436–442.
8. Hosoda K, Yasuda T (1989) Homogeneous immunoassay for alpha 2 plasmin inhibitor (alpha 2-PI) and alpha 2 PI-plasmin complex. J Immun Methods 121: 121–128.
9. Kawakami M, Kawagoe M, Harigai M, Hara M, Hirose T, et al. (1989) Elevated plasma levels of alpha 2 plasmin inhibitor-plasmin complex in patients with rheumatic diseases. Arthr Rheum 32: 1427–1433.

10. Aoki N, Takenaga T, Oguma J, Sumi Y, Koike U, Suzuki H, Hosoda K (1987) Fundamental assessment of enzyme immunoassay kits for alpha 2 plasmin inhibitor (alpha 2 PI) and alpha 2 PI-plasmin complex. Jpn J Clin Pathol 35: 1275-1281.

11. Mimuro J, Koike Y, Sumi Y, Aoki N (1987) Monoclonal antibodies to discrete regions in alpha 2 plasmin inhibitor. Blood 69: 446-453.

12. Saito K, Ito H, Hasegawa T, Yamamoto S (1989) Plasmin alpha 2 plasmin inhibitor complex and α_2-plasmin inhibitor in chronic subdural hematoma. J Neurosurg 70: 68-72.

13. Takahashi Y, Kihara K, Saitoh J, Murai Y, Mori M (1990) Alpha 2 plasmin inhibitor plasmin complex in patients undergone an operation for neck fracture. Clin Path 38: 208-211.

14. Tomiya T, Hayashi S, Ogata I, Fujiwara K (1989) Plasma alpha 2 plasmin inhibitor-plasmin complex and FDP-D-dimer in fulminant hepatic failure. Thromb Resear 53: 253-260.

15. Dudziak R, Kirchhoff PG, Reuter HD, Schumann F (1985) Proteolyse und Proteinaseninhibition in der Herz- und Gefässchirurgie. Stuttgart: FK Schattauer.

16. Jochum M, Dittmer H, Fritz H (1987) Der Effekt des Proteinaseninhibitors Aprotinin auf die Freisetzung granulozytärer Proteinasen und Plasma-proteinveränderungen im traumatisch-hämorrhagischen Schock. Lab Med 11: 235-243.

17. Mosher DF (1990) Blood coagulation and fibrinolysis: an overview. Clin Cardiol 13:VI-5-11.

18. Gonias SL, Figler NL, Braund LL (1988) Regulation of streptokinase-human plasmin complex by the plasma proteinase inhibitor alpha 2 antiplasmin and alpha 2 macroglobulin is species specific and temperature dependent. Blood 72: 1658-1664.

19. Fritz H, Wunderer G (1983) Biochemistry and applications of aprotinin, the kallikrein inhibitor from bovine organs. Arzneimittelforschung 33: 479-494.

20. Royston D (1990) Aprotinin in open-heart surgery: background and results in patients having aortocoronary bypass grafts. Perfusion 5: 63-72.

21. Fraedrich G, Weber C, Bernard C, Hettwer A, Schlosser V (1989) Reduction of blood transfusion requirement in open heart surgery by administration of high doses of aprotinin – preliminary results. Thorac Cardiovasc Surg 37: 89-91.

22. Bidstrup BP, Royston D, Sapsford RN, Taylor KM (1989) Reduction in blood loss and blood use after cardiopulmonary bypass with high dose aprotinin (Trasylol). J Thorac Cardiovasc Surg 97: 364-372.

23. Oeveren W van, Harder MP, Roozendaal KJ, Eijsman L, Wildevuur CRH (1990) Aprotinin protects platelets against the initial effect of cardiopulmonary bypass. J Thorac Cardiovasc Surg 99: 788-797.

24. Oeveren W van, Jansen NJG, Bidstrup BP, et al. (1987) Effects of aprotinin on hemostatic mechanisms during cardiopulmonary bypass. Ann Thorac Surg 44: 640-645.

25. Royston D, Bidstrup BP, Taylor KM, Sapsford RN (1987) Effect of aprotinin on need for blood transfusion after repeat open-heart surgery. Lancet 5: 1289-1291.

26. Dietrich W, Spannagl M, Jochum M, Wendt P, Schramm W, et al. (1990) Influence of high-dose aprotinin treatment on blood loss and coagulation patterns in patients undergoing myocardial revascularization. Anesthesist 73: 1119-1126.

27. Seitz R, Egbring R, Radtke KP, Wolf M, Fuchs G, Fischer J, Lerch L, Karges HE (1985) The clinical significance of alpha 2 antitripsin-elastase and alpha 2 antiplasmin-plasmin complexes for the differentiation of coagulation protein turnover. Int J Tissue React 7: 321-328.

Assessment of mitral regurgitation by color Doppler flow mapping

Steven M. Rosenthal, Navin C. Nanda and Tuong B. Van

Division of Cardiovascular Disease, University of Alabama Medical Center, Birmingham, AL, U.S.A.

Introduction

Conventional Doppler techniques have greatly expanded the capabilities of echocardiography and provide an accurate means of detecting valvular regurgitation. Yet quantification of the regurgitation is difficult and often inaccurate given the great care necessary to detect the flows, the length of time required to do so, and the often eccentric flow patterns. Color Doppler has vastly enhanced conventional pulsed Doppler techniques by increasing the amount and distribution of data that can be collected and instantaneously displayed as a color analogue of blood flow superimposed practically in real time on the two-dimensional image. The ability to visualize the 'color'-coded blood flow has greatly increased our appreciation of the complexity of regurgitant jets, has facilitated the detection of valvular regurgitation and has expanded our ability to assess the severity of regurgitation in a semi-quantitative manner.

Assessment of mitral regurgitation

Mitral regurgitation is a very common abnormality and the mitral valve apparatus is a complex system consisting of the anterior and posterior leaflets, the annular region, the chordae, and the papillary muscles. Their interaction to maintain hemodynamic integrity is poorly understood, although damage to any one part of this system will produce varying levels of valvular insufficiency. Color Doppler allows the detection of valvular insufficiency with great sensitivity and specificity and can be used to semi-quantitate it as well as do existing angiographic methods.

Color Doppler flow reveals the presence of mitral regurgitation as a jet that 'black-flows' from the ventricle across the valve to the atrium. Generally, the size of the jet is determined by the size of the valvular defect and by the transvalvular atrioventricular gradient driving the regurgitant fraction [1]; given the usually large pressure gradient the resultant velocities often exceed the Nyquist limit, producing turbulent jets which are usually easily seen with the appropriate transducer angulation. Recently, in vitro work has also demonstrated that there is a very strong negative correlation between receiving chamber pressure and volume and the size of the regurgitant jet at static compliance; work in a pulsatile system where the effect may even be stronger needs to be pursued [2]. Flow acceleration or convergence often appears on the ventricular side of the regurgitant mitral valve; this occurs as the blood flow converges immediately before it passes through the constricted opening of the leak, and is characterized by a high-velocity laminar flow signal on the ventricular side of the valve immediately distal to the site of leakage. Recognition of this region allows identification of the exact site of regurgitation and may, for instance, allow differentiation of a partially dehisced suture line requiring a relatively simple suture repair from a grossly defective valve requiring a valve repair or replacement.

Performing the examination
The detection and assessment of mitral regurgitation is performed by visualizing the regurgitant jet signals. In order to detect and semi-quantify the jet with color Doppler, it is essential to view it in the plane which best exposes its maximal size. This involves starting the examination with views in each of the three traditional orthogonal planes (the long axis, short axis, and 4-chamber view). Since the largest jet may be moving in a plane intermediate to these, it is necessary to sweep through as many of these planes as possible to find the specific plane in which the area of the jet is maximal. The examination must be performed carefully, since small changes in transducer angulation can produce marked variations in the size of the regurgitant jet, yet it is possible to completely assess the extent of regurgitation in a fraction of the time required by conventional Doppler alone.

Semi-quantification of mitral regurgitation
A variety of measures including the maximum jet length and width have been evaluated, but it is the jet area which provides clinically useful information [3,4]. The jet is first outlined by the operator and then the area of the regurgitant jet is quantified by the onboard computer. The regurgitant jet area can then be expressed as a ratio to left atrial area (measured in the same frame as the maximum jet area) in order to take into account the size of the left atrium, or alternatively, it can be expressed as an absolute size (Table 1). In the first case, using orthogonal transthoracic views of the heart, Helmcke et al. indeed demonstrated that there was a 100% correlation between color Doppler and contrast angiography for the detection of mitral regurgitation in 65 patients who were free of mitral regurgitation and in 82 patients who demonstrated regurgita-

Table 1. Assessment of severity of mitral regurgitation

	Jet area/LA area (%)	Jet area (cm^2)
Mild	< 20	< 4
Moderate	20–40	4–8
Severe	> 40	> 8

tion [3]. Furthermore, they found that the largest jet area to left atrial area ratio could be utilized to semi-quantify the severity of the regurgitation. Briefly, they found that the ratio was less than 0.2 in 34/36 patients with angiographic grade I mitral regurgitation, between 0.2 and 0.4 in 17 of 18 patients with grade II mitral regurgitation, and greater than 0.4 in 26 of 28 patients with grade III regurgitation. Interobserver variability was excellent, with a 0.99 coefficient of correlation between 2 independent observers measuring the regurgitant jet area in the long axis view. Thus, color Doppler flow equalled angiography for reliable detection of mitral regurgitation and for its semi-quantification.

Alternatively, another study of 47 patients reported that the absolute area alone of the maximum regurgitant jet correlated best in their hands with angiographic grading [4]; they noted that < 4 cm^2, 4–8 cm^2, and > 8 cm^2 were the measures which best differentiated mitral regurgitation grades I, II, and III respectively. Small jets less than 0.5 × 2.0 cm could be assigned grade < 1, or 'minimal' regurgitation [5]. It is of course unclear whether a jet in a small left atrium is more or less equivalent to an identically sized jet in a large left atrium.

The assessment of mitral regurgitation can be facilitated by examination of the pulmonary veins for directionality of flow; the venous flow is detected with the color Doppler and the directionality clarified with the pulse wave probe. In the case of severe mitral regurgitation, there will be reversal of flow during systole which should be easily detected. However, unlike the experience with transesophageal echocardiography, the pulmonary veins are not easily identified by the transthoracic approach in most patients with mitral regurgitation.

Although both color Doppler and angiography effectively distinguish clinically severe from mild regurgitation, neither color Doppler [3,4] nor angiography [6] correlates well with the regurgitant fraction calculated from cardiac catheterization indices; however, regurgitant fraction calculated by catheterization and angiography has significant limitations, is not reliable and cannot be considered as a 'gold standard'. Current in vitro research is focussing on calculating the regurgitant fraction from indices measured from the area and velocity of flow convergence [7], but this is difficult to do clinically, since the color Doppler measurements are dependent on the Nyquist limit used. Nevertheless, the absolute jet area or the jet area to left atrial area ratio measured by color Doppler flow mapping is very accurate, especially if the jets are not eccentric, and has become one of the clinical mainstays of assessing the severity of regurgitation. Its sensitivity and specificity are high, generally in the range 80–100%.

Color Doppler assessment of mitral regurgitation due to left ventricular dysfunction
Color Doppler has also been found useful in echocardiographic assessment of mitral regurgitation due to left ventricular dysfunction. It can enhance exercise echocardiography by detecting mitral insufficiency induced by myocardial ischemia. Both isometric [8] and isotonic [9] exercise color Doppler flow mapping have been used in the past to identify ischemia-induced mitral

regurgitation which might otherwise not be apparent. Color Doppler has also been applied in our institution to the detection of mitral regurgitation as a marker for cardiac transplant rejection [10]. Development of new mitral regurgitation or a significant increase in the size of the regurgitant jet heralds the onset of cardiac allograft rejection and correlates fairly well with a positive biopsy showing extensive myocyte necrosis. Disappearance or decrease in the mitral regurgitant jet area is associated with resolution of the rejection process. These color Doppler findings do not correlate well with the severity of allograft rejection but are nevertheless clinically useful in the management of cardiac transplant patients.

Transesophageal echocardiographic assessment
Epicardial and more specifically transesophageal echocardiography have greatly expanded the use of echocardiography and have helped in the assessment of mitral regurgitation in patients with poor transthoracic acoustic windows. The transesophageal approach provides a far superior window for visualization of the heart and the transducers are capable of high-resolution biplane echocardiographic views. Although the geometry of the transesophageal approach limits transducer movement so that the apical and left atrial views may be foreshortened, thus rendering left atrial measurement inaccurate, excellent views can still be obtained; furthermore, many intermediate nonconventional planes can be generated which would be expected to provide a more comprehensive evaluation of the mitral regurgitant jet. The transesophageal approach enables a very detailed study of the mitral valve structure; it is now possible to examine the valvular pathology in minute detail, and to determine the source of the regurgitation with greater precision. Yoshida et al. [11] using biplane transesophageal echocardiography noted excellent levels of sensitivity, in the range 80–100%, for the detection of the varying grades of insufficiency. Despite some data overlap, they felt that angiographically determined mild mitral regurgitation generally demonstrated a maximum jet area of 1.5–4.0 cm^2, while moderate and severe regurgitation produced jet areas between 4.0 and 7.0 cm^2, and greater than 7.0 cm^2, respectively. They also found that mitral regurgitant jets smaller than 1.5 cm^2 were not associated with detectable regurgitation by angiography.

In contrast to the difficulty of evaluating pulmonary venous flow with transthoracic echocardiography, the transesophageal approach provides easy detection of pulmonary flow Doppler signals. As noted previously, the occurrence of systolic flow reversal signifies severe mitral regurgitation, in our experience.

In addition to allowing much improved visualization and functional assessment of native as well as prosthetic valves, transesophageal echocardiography has also enabled the performance of intraoperative echocardiography and routinely provides immediate feedback to the cardiovascular surgeons regarding the efficacy of mitral valve repair. Currently, preoperative assessment can be performed which very accurately details the site of origin of mitral regurgitation, its maximum size as well as the status of the other valves and chamber function; and then, during the intraoperative procedure, it is possible to quickly delineate the results of the mitral valve reapir so that if excessive regurgitation persists, of excessive functional stenosis occurs secondary to the repair, it is possible to correct the repair or replace the valve prior to closing the chest, thus reducing the need for a second operation. Reichert et al. [12] and Kleinman et al. [13] have reported excellent sensitivity for the detection of mitral regurgitation in this setting.

Limitations

A variety of technical factors can affect the use of color Doppler techniques. As is the case with conventional Doppler, color Doppler cannot be used effectively in the absence of adequate-quality two-dimensional echocardiographic images, although generally it is possible to obtain these in the great majority of patients for clinical purposes. Improper machine settings can significantly affect the size of the regurgitant jet. For instance, inadequate gain may cause severe underestimation of the jet size, while excessive gain makes it difficult to delineate the regurgitant jet. Since the Doppler beam often has to traverse the heart longitudinally from the apex through the atria, the Doppler signals can become attenuated, and therefore it is advisable to use a lower-frequency transducer which provides less optimal two-dimensional image resolution but higher penetration capability and improved quality color Doppler signals. Typically, a 2.0 or 2.5 MHz transducer is used for assessment of mitral regurgitation in the clinical setting.

There are several patient-related problems that can alter the assessment of mitral regurgitation. These include low cardiac output and hypotension, which will reduce the atrioventricular pressure gradient, resulting in visibly less regurgitation even though there may actually be severe valve complex related damage. A powerful eccentric jet may lose its energy prematurely as it hits a side wall and appear less significant than it is. Finally, a large leaflet vegetation can affect the penetration of the ultrasonic beam, causing attenuation of the energy of the regurgitant flow. Alternatively, increased afterload caused by systemic hypertension, aortic valve stenosis, or obstructive cardiomyopathy will exaggerate the atrioventricular gradient and regurgitant area. Mitral valve prolapse or chordae rupture with its usually eccentric jets can result in underestimation of regurgitation [14], or conversely overestimation of the regurgitation if it is not recognized that the majority of regurgitation in some patients with mitral valve prolapse may occur only during part of systole (Table 2). Nevertheless, these are usually easily managed problems in experienced hands; for example, in patients with eccentric jets, it is routine to add a grade to the one estimated from jet area to left atrial area ratio. In our hands, if a markedly eccentric regurgitation was felt to be moderate on the basis of calculating the jet area/left atrial area ratio, it would be reported as severe (grade III).

Table 2.

Causes of underestimation of mitral regurgitation

1. Poor transthoracic acoustic window.
2. Low cardiac output/hypotension.
3. Eccentric jet (impaction against wall) such as with mitral valve prolapse and chordae rupture.
4. Large leaflet vegetation.
5. Improper machine settings.

Causes of overestimation of mitral regurgitation

1. Mitral valve prolapse with mid to late systolic mitral regurgitation.
2. Systemic hypertension.
3. Aortic valve stenosis/left ventricular outflow tract obstruction.

Conclusion

In conclusion, color Doppler has greatly improved our ability to detect and semi-quantify mitral regurgitation. Although we cannot precisely calculate the regurgitant fraction, color Doppler allows accurate description of the regurgitant jet and permits us to distinguish severe from mild or clinically insignificant mitral regurgitation. For the surgeon's benefit, transesophageal echocardiography with color Doppler facilitates intraoperative assessment of the status of all the cardiac valves and can be used to reliably notify the surgeon regarding the adequacy of valve repair in time to permit revisions prior to closing the chest.

References

1. Switzer DF, Yoganathan AP, Nanda NC, Woo YR, Ridgway AJ (1985) Circulation 72: III–207 (abstr).
2. Maciel BC, Moises VA, Shandas R, Simpson IA, Beltran M, Valdes-Cruz L, Sahn D (1991) Circulation 83: 605–613.
3. Helmcke F, Nanda NC, Hsiung MC, Soto B, Adey C, Goyal RG, Gatewood RP Jr (1987) Circulation 75: 175–182.
4. Spain MG, Smith MD, Harrison M, Grayburn P, Kwan OL, O'Brien M, DeMaria AN (1989) J Am Coll Cardiol 13: 585–590.
5. Cooper JW, Nanda NC, Fan PH (1990) In: LP Zipes and DJ Rowlands, eds. Progress in Cardiology 3/1. Philadelphia: Lea and Febiger 67–81.
6. Croft CH, Lipscomb K, Mathis K, Firth BG, Nicod P, Tilton G, Winniford MD, Hills LD (1984) Am J Cardiol 53: 1593–1598.
7. Recusani F, Bargiggia GS, Yoganathan AP, Raisaro A, Valdes-Cruz LM, Sung HW, Bertucci C, Gallati M, Moises VA, Simpson IA Tronconi L, Sahn DJ (1991) Circulation 83: 594–603.
8. Zachariah ZP, Hsiung MC, Nanda NC, Kan MN, Gatewood RP Jr (1987) Am J Cardiol 59: 166–170.
9. Spain MG, Smith MD, Kwan OL, DeMaria AN (1990) Am J Cardiol 65: 78–83.

10. Hsiung MC, Nanda NC, Kirklin JK, Bittner V, Smith S (1986) Circulation 74: IV-132.
11. Yoshida K, Yoshikawa J, Yamaura Y, Hozumi T, Akasaki T, Fukaya T (1990) Circulation 82: 1121-1126.
12. Reichert SLA, Visser CA, Moulijn AC, Suttorp MJ, vd Brink RBA, Koolen JJ, Jaarsma W, Vereulen F, Dunning AJ (1990) J Thorac Cardiovasc Surg 100: 756-761.
13. Kleinman JP, Czer LSC, DeRobertis M, Chaux A, Maurer G (1989) G Am J Cardiol 64: 1168-1172.
14. Wilcox I, Fletcher PJ, Bailey BP (1989) Eur Heart J 10: 872-879.

Decision-making by transcutaneous and transesophageal Doppler color flow mapping followed by intraoperative direct scanning in dissecting aortic aneurysm

Shinichi Takamoto[1], Shunei Kyo[2], Yuji Yokote[2] and Ryozo Omoto[2]

[1]Division of Cardiovascular Surgery, Showa General Hospital, Kodaira, Tokyo 187 and
[2]Department of Surgery, Saitama Medical School, Saitama 350-04, Japan

Introduction

Since dissecting aortic aneurysm is a serious disorder which may be fatal soon after onset, early and accurate diagnosis is mandatory for saving lives. Recently a clinical application of Doppler color flow mapping has become widespread in the field of cardiovascular medicine. In the field of diagnosis of dissecting aortic aneurysm we first applied conventional transcutaneous color flow mapping in 1948 [1]. In 1985 we first reported intraoperative color flow mapping in the surgery of this disease [2], and in 1986 we first applied transesophageal color flow mapping to the visualization of thoracic dissecting aortic aneurysm where high-quality images and accurate diagnosis could not be obtained with conventional transcutaneous approaches [3,4]. We have proposed that these modalities of color flow mapping, transcutaneous and transesophageal color flow mapping followed by intraoperative scanning, will provide sufficiently accurate and quick information to guide decision-making in the treatment of this severe disorder even without aortography. The purpose of this paper is to evaluate the clinical significance of this strategy for aortic dissection, decision-making by transcutaneous and transesophageal color flow mapping followed by intraoperative scanning in 67 cases.

Material and Methods

Sixty-seven cases of dissecting aortic aneurysm admitted to Saitama Medical School and Showa General Hospital from October 1985 to April 1991 and examined by the first author were investigated. The patients were 45 males and 22 females, and mean age was 59.3 ± 13.4 yr.

Thirty-five acute and 32 chronic cases were included. DeBakey type differentiation was 15 cases of type I, 7 cases of type II, 34 cases of type III, 5 cases of type III with retrograde dissection (III R), one case of type II + III, 2 cases of postoperative state of former type I, 3 cases of postoperative state of former type III. Within the 67 cases surgery was performed in 31 cases and intraoperative scanning was done in 30 cases.

The equipment used in this study was the Aloka 880, 870, 340 color flow mapping system utilizing a 3.5 or 5.0 MHz transducer, which was gas-sterilized for intraoperative direct scanning. The transesophageal probes used were Aloka's transverse scanning, longitudinal scanning and bi-plane scanning probes, which have an ultrasound frequency of 5.0 MHz.

Our strategies for acute dissecting aortic aneurysms are shown in Fig. 1. Patients who are suspected of acute dissection are admitted to the intensive care unit, and a routine examination which includes chest and abdominal X-ray, ECG and blood analysis is done. Then transcutaneous echocardiography is performed utilizing various approaches to the aorta which include conventional transthoracic approaches through right and left parasternal and suprasternal windows, and the cervical approaches to the arch vessels and abdominal approaches to the abdominal aorta. If suspicion of dissection still remains, the transesophageal transducer is swallowed with local anesthesia of the throat. Transesophageal echocardiography examination with color flow mapping can differentiate DeBakey type of dissection. If it is type III without severe complications such as rupture or organ ischemia, the patient goes to the medical treatment program. If the patient is diagnosed as type I or II or III R or type III with such complications and is operable with regard to general condition, emergent surgery is prepared and performed. During surgery intraoperative direct scanning is performed for intraoperative decision-making and evaluation of the postoperative state. After surgery transcutaneous and mainly transesophageal color flow mapping are performed for follow-up of the patient.

In chronic dissection, which allows much time for preparation, aortography with coronary angiogram is usually performed with a transesophageal echocardiography study. If a dissection is type I, II, III R or type III with enlarged aorta whose diameter extends over 6 cm, elective surgery is performed with intraoperative direct scanning used as a guide.

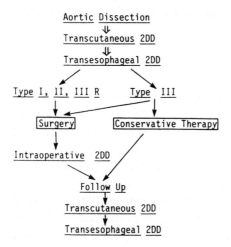

Fig. 1. Strategy of decision-making for acute aortic dissection. 2DD, 2-D Doppler color flow mapping.

Results

Areas covered by transcutaneous, transesophageal and intraoperative scanning (Fig. 2)
Transcutaneous echo definitely imaged the area of the heart and the aortic root by the left parasternal approach and the carotid artery by the cervical approach, and occasionally imaged the area of the upper ascending aorta by the right parasternal approach, the aortic arch by the suprasternal approach, and the abdominal aorta and the abdominal branches by the abdominal approach. An almost absolute blind spot for transcutaneous echo was the descending aorta.

Transesophageal echo imaged the whole descending aorta, the heart and the proximal ascending aorta definitely and the upper abdominal aorta occasionally. Longitudinal scan imaged the aortic arch and the arch vessels frequently. A blind spot for transesophageal echo was the upper ascending aorta.

Intraoperative echo definitely imaged the heart and the ascending aorta and the aortic arch through median sternotomy and the heart and the whole thoracic aorta through left lateral thoracotomy. Intraoperative echo through mini-laparotomy definitely imaged the whole abdominal aorta and the iliac arteries, while intraoperative transcutaneous echo only occasionally displayed those regions.

Transcutaneous color flow mapping
Diagnosis of dissection was made by detection of an intimal flap in the aorta. Transcutaneous color flow mapping revealed an intimal flap in any portion of the aorta and could diagnose dissection in 54 cases (81%) out of 67 cases, while transesophageal color flow mapping could diagnose dissection in all 67 cases (100%). Transcutaneous approach could not reveal an intimal flap in 13 cases

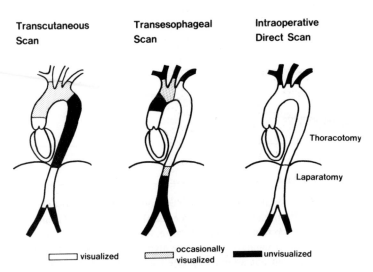

Fig. 2. Visualization of the aorta by echo examination.

(19%), which consisted of 3 of type II, 9 of type III and one of type III with retrograde dissection (III R), DeBakey type differentiation was impossible due to a lack of clarity in the range of involved dissection in the aorta.

Transesophageal color flow mapping

Site of the initial entry was detected in 52 cases (78%) by transesophageal color flow mapping but undetected in 15 cases (22%), which included 7 of type I, 5 of type II, 2 of type III, and one of type III R (Table 1). However, differentiation of DeBakey type was performed correctly in 65 cases (97%). Only 2 cases (3%) which were misdiagnosed as type I because of failure to detect the initial entry at the ascending aorta were changed in diagnosis to type II + III, and type III R during the surgery, respectively (Table 2). Differentiation of DeBakey type was based on hemodynamics in the false lumen in 14 cases out of 15 cases in which the initial entry was undetected by transesophageal color flow mapping (Fig. 3). In 2 cases transcutaneous right parasternal approach could depict it and intraoperative scanning displayed it in eight operative cases.

Aortic regurgitation was displayed in 21 cases by transesophageal color flow mapping and graded by the distance of the regurgitant jet. Three of grade 1, 12 of grade 2 and 6 of grade 3 were displayed. Resuspension of aortic valve was performed in 5 cases and postoperative grading of aortic regurgitation was confirmed in grade 1 in all operative cases.

Complete thrombus formation in the false lumen was displayed in 6 cases (16%), one of type I and 5 of type III. In one case of type III R complete

Table 1. Detection of site of the initial entry by transesophageal echo

Detected		52		(78%)
Undectected		15		(22%)
	I		7	
	II		5 (1)	
	III		2	
	III R		1 (1)	

( ): type differentiation incorrect.

Table 2. Differentiation of DeBakey type by transesophageal echo

Correct	65 (97%)
Incorrect	2

Fig. 3. Hemodynamics in the true (TL) and false lumens (FL) at the aortic arch by transesophageal color flow mapping. A forward flow (from the proximal to the distal) in systole in TL and FL indicated an entry at the more proximal portion (see opposite page, top).

Fig. 4. The transesophageal longitudinal scanning images of the arch vessels. Note that an entry (En) is shown at the level of the brachiocephalic artery. LSCA, left subclavian artery; LCCA, left common carotid artery; BCA, brachiocephalic artery (see opposite page, bottom).

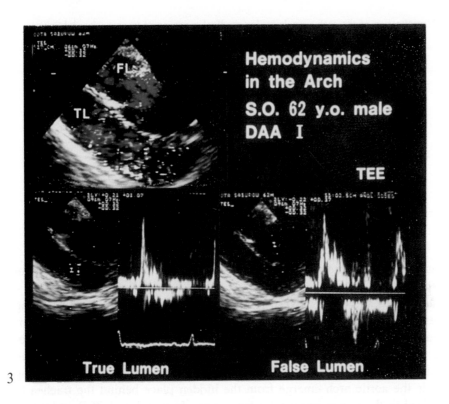

3

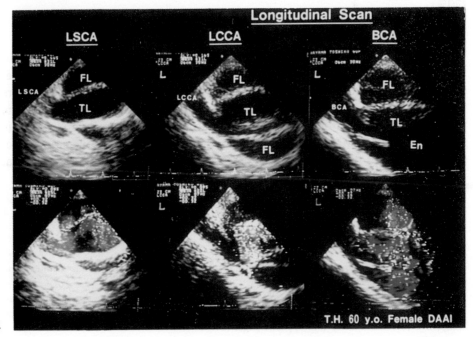

4

Table 3. Visualization of the arch vessels by longitudinal scanning of transesophageal echo

	Visualization	Dissection
Total	42 cases	
LSCA	40 (95%)	6 (15%)
LCCA	25 (59%)	2 (9%)
BCA	16 (38%)	7 (43%)
Type I & III R	15 cases	
LSCA	15 (100%)	4 (26%)
LCCA	11 (73%)	2 (18%)
BCA	10 (66%)	7 (70%)

LSCA, left subclavian artery; LCCA, left common carotid artery; BCA, brachiocephalic artery.

thrombus formation in the ascending aorta was displayed and medical treatment was selected.

The aortic arch and the arch vessels were examined by longitudinal scanning of transesophageal color flow mapping in 42 patients (Table 3) (Fig. 4). The left subclavian artery was well visualized in all types of dissection. The brachiocephalic artery and the left common carotid artery were visualized in 66% and 73%, respectively, in type I and III R. Involvement of dissection to the ascending aorta made the aortic arch emerge from the hidden place behind the trachea to be visualized in the transesophageal echo images. In type I and III R, extension of dissection to the brachiocephalic artery was relatively high in 7 out of 10 (70%).

Intraoperative scanning
Intraoperative scanning was performed in 30 patients: 8 of type I, 5 of type II, 9 of type III, 3 of type III R, 1 of type II + III, 2 of postoperative state of former type I and 2 of postoperative state of former type III. Ascending aortic procedure was performed in 15 cases, aortic arch procedure in 6 cases, descending aortic procedure in 5 cases, thoraco-abdominal procedure in 2 cases, abdominal aortic procedure in one case and ligation of the left subclavian artery in one case. Direct scanning of color flow mapping was performed in 29 cases and transesophageal scanning was performed in 2 cases. (In one case both scannings were done.) Direct scanning was done through median sternotomy in 16 cases and through left lateral thoracotomy in 12 cases and through laparotomy in one case. In 4

Fig. 5. Intraoperative direct scanning images at the ascending aorta of DeBakey type I. An entry (arrow) which was not detected by transesophageal echo was imaged clearly by this scanning, and the precise operative procedure was determined (see opposite page, top).
Fig. 6. Intraoperative direct scanning images of the abdominal aortic branches through mini-laparatomy. All branches have sufficient flow. SMA, superior mesenteric artery; RRA, right renal artery; LRA, left renal artery (see opposite page, bottom).

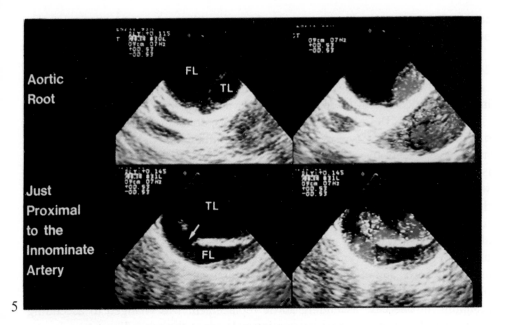

5

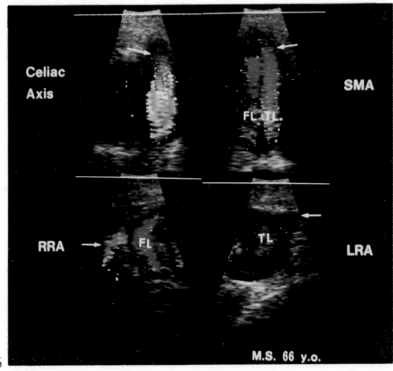

6

cases of thoracotomy direct scanning through additional mini-laparotomy was performed.

Size and site of the initial entry were confirmed by intraoperative scanning in 29 cases (97%). Flow states in the true and false lumina were visualized in all cases (100%). In 15 cases thrombus in the false lumen was visualized. This information was useful to decide the site of aortic clamp.

Correction of DeBakey type diagnosis was done in 2 cases. Preoperative diagnosis of DeBakey type was confirmed by intraoperative color flow mapping in all cases except two, in which preoperative diagnosis type I was corrected to type II + III with true aortic arch aneurysm and type III R. Extent of dissection was corrected in one case, in which type I dissection was found to extend from the distal aortic arch to the abdomen. In eight cases the initial entry was newly found in intraoperative direct scanning, although transesophageal scanning had already suggested the site of the initial entry by the hemodynamics in the false lumen (Fig. 5). In seven cases the newly found initial entry existed in the ascending aorta, and in one case it was at the left subclavian artery. In three cases planned surgical procedures were changed based on the information from direct scanning; in one case ascending aortic replacement was changed to ascending aortoplasty because of the transverse intimal tear at the ascending aorta; in one case ascending aortic replacement was changed to ascending-arch aortic replacement because the entry was visualized at the innominate artery level by direct scanning; in the third case aortic arch replacement was planned at first; however, intraoperative echo indicated an entry at the left subclavian artery, and the surgery performed was simply ligation of the left subclavian artery (Table 4).

Precise surgical procedure, site and direction of the aortic incision and extent of the graft replacement were determined in all cases based on the information provided by intraoperative direct scanning of color flow mapping. During cardiopulmonary bypass safe perfusion in the aorta from the bypass was confirmed by intraoperative color flow mapping in 20 cases; in one case re-dissection was confirmed. Site of occlusion balloon catheter in the descending aorta was confirmed in two cases.

Supplemental diagnostic laparotomy, involving a direct scanning of color flow mapping to the abdominal aorta and vessels (Fig. 6) and the iliac artery, was performed in 4 cases. In the case of type II + III, dissection was shown to extend into the superior mesenteric artery by intraoperative echo, and ischemia of the intestine was driven. After the main procedure was done, fenestration of the superior mesenteric artery was performed. The iliac artery was examined by intraoperative echo through mini-laparotomy to determine the cannulation side at the femoral artery. A contralateral side of the dissected iliac artery was selected for cannulation.

After the vascular procedure was finished, flow dynamics in the true and false lumen were visualized in all cases. Flow in the false lumen was visualized in 7 cases, which meant leakage from the anastomosis or existence of the entry near the anastomosis, and no flow in the false lumen was visualized in 17 cases. In

Table 4. Results of intraoperative scanning in 30 cases in the prevascular clamp state

Confirmation	
Initial tear	29 (97%)
Flow state in two lumens	30 (100%)
Thrombus in the false lumen	15
Safe perfusion from pump	20
Re-dissection	1
Site of occlusion balloon	2
Correction	
DeBakey type diagnosis	2
I → II + III	1
I → III R	1
Extent of dissection	1
Changes of surgical procedure	3
Asc Ao replacement →	Plasty
Asc Ao replacement →	Asc-Arch Ao replacement
Arch Ao replacement →	Ligation of LSCA

Asc Ao, ascending aorta; LSCA, left subclavian artery.

6 cases the false lumen was completely resected. Leakage from the suture line was visualized in 3 cases. In one case additional sutures were done.

Results of surgery
Of the 31 cases 14 were acute and 17 chronic. Early operative death occurred in 5 acute cases and one chronic case. In the acute cases causes of death were infection in 2 cases and brain damage in 2 cases and intestinal ischemia due to late embolization in one case. In the chronic cases one death was caused by graft versus host disease. These outcomes were not related to decision-making based on transesophageal or intraoperative echo.

In the 14 acute cases, 4 cases were examined by aortography as well, but on reflection we found that aortography could be bypassed in this decision-making.

Discussion

Color flow mapping has resulted in great progress in the noninvasive diagnosis of cardiovascular diseases. However, there is difficulty in obtaining images of the entire thoracic aorta by transcutaneous color flow mapping due to poor penetration of echo in the thorax. Transcutaneous echo windows to the aorta are limited in the chest and the abdomen, and moreover the air in the thorax and the bowel may inhibit echo penetration. If it can depict the intimal flap in any region of the aorta, diagnosis of the aortic dissection can be obtained but not type differentiation as in our series.

Recently we have reported that transesophageal color flow mapping was useful to display dissection of the thoracic aorta [4,5]. However, transesophageal echo itself has shortcomings in the visualization of the whole thoracic aorta; that is, the upper ascending aorta and sometimes the aortic arch are poorly visualized due to the inhibition of echo penetration by the trachea intervening between the aorta and the esophagus.

In our series the initial entry was not visualized by transesophageal echo in 22% of the cases. However, even without direct visualization of the initial entry hemodynamics in the false lumen can supply rough information of the site and size of the initial entry. Therefore, DeBakey type differentiation can be obtained by transesophageal color flow mapping in almost al cases (97%). If DeBakey type differentiation is determined, the surgical approaches, median sternotomy or lateral thoracotomy, can be decided. If a case is type I, II or III R without complete thrombus formation in the false lumen in the ascending aorta, median sternotomy will be performed. If a case is type III with serious complications such as rupture or organ ischemia, lateral thoracotomy will be performed in emergency surgery. This decision is sometimes difficult if only transverse scanning with transesophageal echo is performed in a case of dissection in which an entry exists at the arch and the aortic arch is involved by dissection. However, as shown in Table 3, in type I or III R the aortic arch is relatively easily visualized and evaluated by transesophageal longitudinal scanning.

Even after the emergency surgery is started, there remain blind spots in the region of the upper ascending aorta and the aortic arch which transesophageal echo may not visualize. Intraoperative direct scanning using a sterile transducer displays vividly these regions. Intraoperative direct scanning not only supplements the preoperative diagnosis by transesophageal echo but also determines the precise and most appropriate operative procedure. The site of the aortic incision, site of the aortic clamp, range of the graft replacement, graft replacement or simple closure of the entry are all determined finally by intraoperative direct scanning.

During surgery of dissecting aortic aneurysm, cardiopulmonary bypass is usually employed, and difficulty of perfusion through the cannula is occasionally encountered. Intraoperative echo clearly demonstrates the perfusion status in both the true and the false lumina and indicates safe perfusion. In our series we have encountered a case of re-dissection due to retrograde perfusion through the femoral artery. Intraoperative echo displayed three lumens with a dilated, newly dissected lumen.

To obtain safe perfusion of cardiopulmonary bypass, it is important to decide the cannulation site of the femoral artery to the non-dissected artery. Although information on extension of dissection to the iliac artery is needed, it is sometimes difficult to obtain even by aortography because of the remote position from the main interest area. Transcutaneous echo may supply that information. If not, intraoperative echo through mini-laparatomy may give us such information [5]. Mini-laparatomy is easily done in a short time during general anesthesia, and direct scanning through it is very useful if information on the abdominal vessels is not obtained by other methods.

After vascular procedures, intraoperative direct scanning reveals information about flow dynamics in the true and false lumina and the effects of surgery are evaluated. If any defect is found by intraoperative echo through thoracotomy or mini-laparatomy, additional procedures can be performed before chest closure. This method is the only way to evaluate the postoperative status of dissection accurately in the operating room.

Surgery of dissecting aortic aneurysm has a high mortality, especially in acute cases. In our series acute dissections have 36% mortality, and chronic cases have 6%. In our acute series this mortality is related to very severe conditions due to rupture in 3 cases and infection in 2 cases, and is not related to color flow mapping decision-making itself. We believe this technique using transesophageal and intraoperative color flow mapping may improve this severe mortality by providing quick and proper decision-making.

Conclusions

1. In decision-making for aortic dissection using color flow mapping, trans-cutaneous scanning provides rough information on the existence of dissection. Transesophageal scanning permits confirmation of diagnosis of aortic dissection and determination of DeBakey type differentiation and surgical approaches.
2. Intraoperative direct scanning through thoracotomy and mini-laparatomy permits determination of precise operative procedure and evaluation of effects of surgery, compensating for the shortcomings of transesophageal scanning.
3. This combination of three modalities, transcutaneous, transesophageal, and intraoperative direct scanning of color flow mapping, can provide entire images of the aorta and its branches. They can lead to proper and quick decision-making for treatment of aortic dissection, especially for acute cases, even without aortography.

Acknowledgements

This study was supported by grants from the Japan Heart Foundation in 1986, the Mitsui Life Social Welfare Foundation in 1987 and the Japan Medical Association in 1987.

References

1. Takamoto S (1984) In: R Omoto, ed. Color Atlas of Real-Time Two-Dimensional Doppler Echocardiography. Tokyo: Shindan-to-Chiryo, 135–143, 155–160.
2. Takamoto S, Kyo S, Adachi H, et al. (1985) J Thorac Cardiovasc Surg 90: 802–812.
3. Takamoto S, Kyo S, Matsumura M, et al. (1986) Circulation 74 (Suppl II): 132.

4. Takamoto S, Omoto R (1987) Herz 12: 187–193.
5. Takamoto S, Kyo S, Omoto R (1989) In: G Maurer and W Mohl, eds. Echocardiography and Doppler in Cardiac Surgery. New York: Igaku-Shoin, 275–284.

Cardio-thoracic surgery. K. Minami et al. editors.

115

Quantitative color Doppler analysis of shunt/regurgitation volumes in congenital heart disease

H. Meyer, K. Vyska, G. Goerg, W. Matthies and W.R. Thies
Department of Pediatric Cardiology, Heart Centre NRW, Bad Oeynhausen, F.R.G.

Introduction

In the last decade echocardiography became an established part of clinical cardiological diagnosis. It provides valuable morphological information as well as data concerning the local velocities and pressure gradients. The introduction of color Doppler echocardiography (CDE) provides, moreover, qualitative insights into the flow situation in the ventricular cavities. Until now, however, it has not been possible to obtain quantitative information by the use of this technique.

Since a simple non-invasive quantitative assessment of the left to right shunt with congenital septal defects and of regurgitation flow in mitral valve insufficiency would be for a pediatric cardiologist of elementary importance, it was the aim of this study to develop a method which would provide this information by means of the color echocardiographic technique.

Material and Methods

In this study, 60 children with ventricular septal defect and 30 patients with atrial septal defect and left to right systolic shunt as well as 12 children with mitral valve insufficiency were evaluated. The age of the children with ventricular septal defect ranged from 7 days to 16 yr (mean: 12 mth). The weight ranged from 3.3 to 53 kg (mean: 8.4 kg). Each patient had undergone cardiac catheterization, and pulmonary (Qp) as well as systemic (Q_s) blood flow were calculated. The shunt volume (SV) was determined by the Fick method (oxymetrically) and by use of the thermodilution method. The flow velocity in the area of septal defects or at the level of mitral valve was determined by continuous-wave Doppler. With all measurements precautions were taken in order to obtain comparable examination conditions.

Color flow mapping was performed with Ultramark 9 color Doppler. This color Doppler is a 3.5 MHz scanner providing 90° sector images. Color flow mapping was performed over 32 lines across 60° of sector angle, usually at 6 kHz. Frame rate was 15/s over 9 cm depth with Nyquist limits at 66 cm/s. The color table was normalized to the respective Nyquist limit. As the criterion for gain setting the optimal image of aortic flow was used. All Doppler studies were performed in long-axis, short-axis, and four-chamber views. ECG gating was used. Each study was reviewed frame by frame by video play-back to analyse the defects and the flows across the defects. From these images the one with maximal area of the imaged shunt was selected and its area was determined planimetrically. The flow velocity in the area of septal defect was determined by continuous-wave Doppler (CW).

Oximetry

Samples of blood were taken from superior caval vein (SVC) (high and low levels), inferior caval vein (IVC) (level of diaphragm), pulmonary artery (left, right, and main), two samples from pulmonary vein (if foramen ovale was patent) as well as one from arteria femoralis (arterial and pulmonary venous saturations were equal in VSD with LR shunt). Each sample was analyzed for O_2 saturation. The sample run was carried out in 1–2 min and repeated later in the procedure. The O_2 consumption per minute was indexed for body surface area.

The pulmonary blood flow (Q_p) and systemic flow (Q_s) were obtained by applying the Fick principle.

Systemic flow:

$$Q_s = \frac{\dot{V}O_2}{C_aO_2 - C_vO_2}$$

where $\dot{V}O_2$ = oxygen consumption (ml/min), C_aO_2 = arterial O_2 saturation (%), C_vO_2 = mixed venous O_2 saturation, preshunt (%).

The mixed venous O_2 saturation was obtained by equating it to the average of blood O_2 saturation SVC and IVC samples.

Pulmonary flow:

$$Q_p = \frac{\dot{V}O_2}{C_{pv}O_2 - C_{pa}O_2}$$

where $C_{pv}O_2$ = O_2 saturation of pulmonary venous blood (%), $C_{pa}O_2$ saturation of pulmonary arterial blood (%).

Thermodilution technique (measurement of pulmonary blood flow (Q_p))

A thermal indicator (saline) was injected into venae cavae and the resultant change in blood temperature was continuously recorded by a thermistor, mounted on the tip of the catheter (Swan-Ganz catheter Q3-132-SF; Edwards Corp.) at the trunk of the pulmonary artery. The registered data were evaluated by the means of the Schwarzer cardiac-output computer IVF 4000.

Theory

In order to interpret the data obtained by color flow mapping we first considered the hydrodynamic properties of a jet of fluid issuing in the space filled with the same fluid (Fig. 1). The fluid in which the jet expands was considered to be in stationary state. As demonstrated by Landau et al. [1] and Prandtl [2], in such a case the jet region is a cone with a constant opening angle of 25° to 30°. The average axial component of the velocity in the jet, u, was found to decrease with increase of the distance from the apex of the cone. This means that with increasing cone radius the average axial component of the flow velocity decreases.

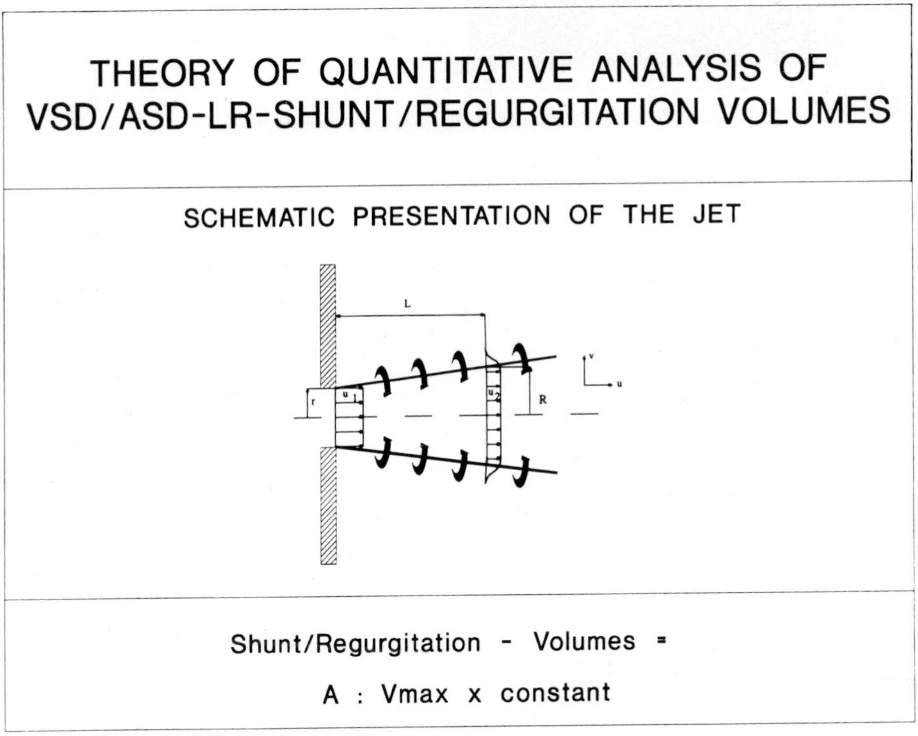

THEORY OF QUANTITATIVE ANALYSIS OF
VSD/ASD-LR-SHUNT/REGURGITATION VOLUMES

SCHEMATIC PRESENTATION OF THE JET

Shunt/Regurgitation - Volumes =

A : Vmax x constant

Fig. 1. Schematic representation of the jet. In this figure u_1 and u_2 are the average axial velocities in cross-sections with radius r and R, respectively. v is the velocity in y-direction. It is practically constant in the cross-section and equals 2.5% of the axial velocity. v is directed into the jet. This velocity component causes the influx of the fluid in the jet 'jet suction'. This means that by the quantitative determination of the shunt volume the flow must be directly determined in the cross-section of the septal defect, where the y-component of the velocity is zero and no effects of jet 'suction' are present.

118

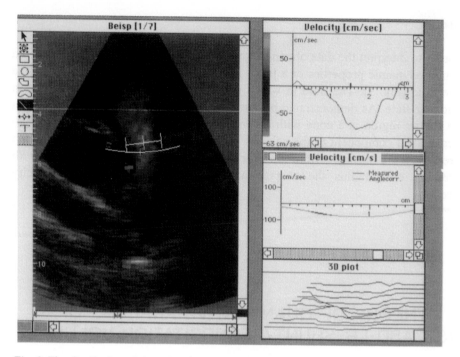

Fig. 2. The distribution of the velocities in a selected cross-section of the jet.

The analysis of the data obtained by the color flow mapping indicated a flat velocity profile in the jet (see Fig. 2).

Under these conditions the dependence of the average axial velocity on the cone radius can be derived by the use of the momentum flux conservation law [1,2]. According to this law the momentum flux in the jet region is constant [1], i.e.

$$r \cdot u_1^2 \cdot r^2 = r \cdot u_2^2 \cdot R^2 \tag{1}$$

where r is the fluid density, and u_1 and u_2 are the average axial velocities in cross-sections with radius r and R, respectively,

After rearranging this relationship one obtains:

$$R = r \cdot u_1/u_2 \tag{2}$$

Since according to Sass et al. [2] and Landau et al. [1] the opening angle of the jet cone is practically constant and equals 25°, the following relationship between R and L can be derived:

$$L = (R - r)/\text{tg}25° \tag{3}$$

where L is distance between cross-sections R and r.

After substitution of eq. (2) into eq. (3) one obtains:

$$L = r \cdot u_1/u_2(1 - u_2/u_1)/tg25° \tag{4}$$

By ultrasound color mapping with color scaling normalized to a fixed maximal velocity the boundary of the jet recognizable by eye corresponds practically always to the same velocity. Let L be the maximal distance of recognizable jet intrusion, then according to eq. (4) the maximal distance of recognizable jet intrusion is to be expected to be a linear function of flow velocity multiplied by the hole diameter r. The validity of this conclusion is demonstrated by the model experiments done by Sugawara et al. [3] and Wranne et al. [4], who studied the distance of intrusion at different driving pressures and different tube diameters.

Since the jet is a cone the area (A) of the jet in the x–y plane between the jet origin and L is given by:

$$A = L \cdot (r + R) \tag{5}$$

After substitution of eqs. (2) and (4) into eq. (5) one obtains:

$$A = r^2 \cdot (u_1/u_2)^2 \cdot (1 - (u_2/u_1)^2)/tg25° \tag{6}$$

Since in most color flow scanners the color table is normalized to the velocity corresponding to a Nyquist limit at a selected pulse-repetition-frequency, the border of the maximal area of the recognizable jet (which is selected by the eye) always corresponds to the same color, i.e. to the same velocity u_2 (i.e. $u_2 =$ const). The analysis of repeated evaluations of a given jet by different observers indicated that the eye selects the border at approximately 20% of the velocity corresponding to a Nyquist limit (NL). Under these conditions the following estimate can be done:

$$u_2^2 = (0.2)^2 \cdot NL^2$$

and

$$(u_2/u_1)^2 = (0.2)^2 \cdot (NL/u_1)^2$$

Since the velocity in VSD usually ranges between 2 and 4 m/s, the ratio NL/u_1 is smaller than 1 and

$$(u_2/u_1)^2 < 0.04$$

This value was negligible when compared to 1.

Under these conditions one obtains:

$$A = r^2 \cdot u_1{}^2 / (\text{tg}25° \cdot u_2{}^2) \tag{7}$$

If it is considered that $r^2 \cdot u_1$ is proportional to the flow in the tube opening (F) and that u_2 is practically constant, then the relationship (7) can be written as follows:

$$A = F \cdot u_1 \cdot \text{const} \tag{8}$$

or

$$F = A/u_1 \cdot \text{const} \tag{9}$$

This means that by a selection of a constant color table and normalization of the image to the Nyquist limit, the flow at the opening of the tube (shunt flow) must be expected to be linearly proportional to the ratio of the maximal recognizable area of the jet, A (maximal area of the imaged shunt), and the average flow velocity in the opening of the tube, u_1 (velocity in the septal defect).

For the determination of the average flow velocity in the area of septal defect the integrated continuous wave (CW) Doppler can be used. By the use of CW Doppler it must be, however, considered that this method provides information about the distribution of average velocities which exists along the CW beam in a tube of a cross-section of about 1 cm^2. According to eq. (2) the maximal of these velocities was considered to represent an average velocity in the area of the septal defect, u_1. Using this value the flow through the tube opening, F, can be calculated from maximal area of the imaged shunt (MAIS) and CW determined average velocity in the septal defect by the use of eq. (9).

Results

In all patients suffering from VSD or ASD the shunts were imaged easily as flow crossing the ventricular septal defect. The flow mapping demonstrated the septal defect orifice much better than a two-dimensional echocardiogram.

Two representative examples of determination of MAIS are shown in Figs. 3 and 4.

Figure 3 demonstrates a color Doppler echocardiography of a 6-mth-old patient with ventricular septal defect. The short axis chamber view demonstrates a perimembraneous VSD. Maximal area of the imaged shunt was 0.21 cm^2/m^2 BS. Maximal velocity was 4 m/s. In this case the imaged shunt has an ideal form. The jet region is a cone. The smaller cross-section corresponds to the septal defect.

In Fig. 4 a color Doppler echocardiography of a 6-mth-old patient with ventricular septal defect can be seen. The parasternal long-axis view demonstrates

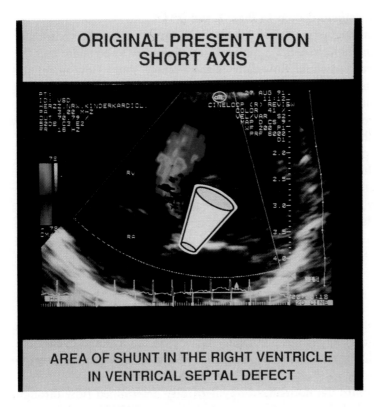

Fig. 3. Color Doppler echocardiography of a 6-mth-old patient A.G. with ventricular septal defect; short axis view demonstrates a perimembraneous VSD. Maximal area of the imaged shunt was 0.85 cm^2/m^2 BS. Maximal velocity was 4 m/s. Transducer frequency 3.5 MHz; repetition rate 6 kHz.

a perimembraneous VSD. Maximal area of the imaged shunt was 2.3 cm^2/m^2 BS. Maximal velocity was 4.4 m/s. In this case the original cone form of the jet was secondarily altered due to the blood flow in the ventricular cavity.

Figure 5 demonstrates the MAIS obtained in a 6-mth-old patient with perimembraneous VSD by the determinations in long-axis, short-axis and four-chamber views. The MAIS determined in a long axis view was 0.70 cm^2/m^2 BS. In the short axis and 4-chamber views it was 0.65 and 0.85 cm^2/m^2 BS.

Figure 6 shows the MAIS obtained in a 6-mth-old infant with perimembraneous VSD by different repetition frequencies. At a repetition frequency of 6 kHz the MAIS was 0.85 cm^2/m^2; at a repetition frequency of 8 kHz it was 0.60 cm^2/m^2.

In Fig. 7 the angular dependency of the MAIS detected in a 6-mth-old infant with perimembraneous VSD is demonstrated. It can be seen that the angle variation of 15° leads to a change of MAIS from 1.05 cm^2/m^2 to 1.15 cm^2/m^2.

The data obtained by the evaluation of the maximal area of the imaged shunt in all patients with ventricular septal defect are compared with the results obtained by cardiac catheterization in Figs. 8 and 9.

In order to compare the oxymetrically determined flow through the ventricular septal defect with the ratio $MAIS/V_{max}$ it was first necessary to consider that the oxymetrically determined shunt flow reflects the average shunt flow under the theoretical conditions in which the blood would be continuously flowing through the septal defect during the whole period of the cardiac cycle. The actual shunt flow is higher since the given shunted volume of blood has to pass the septal defect not during the whole heart revolution, but only during the duration of systole. By means of color flow mapping not the average, but the actual shunt flow is detected. Therefore, to adequately compare the color flow mapping data with the average data obtained oxymetrically a corresponding correction must be done. Consequently, we normalized the oxymetrically determined flow to actual flow by dividing it by the systolic proportion of the cardiac cycle, i.e. the oxymetrically determined flow through the septal defect was normalized to actual flow by use of the following relationship:

$$QP \cdot Q_p \cdot t_c/60 \cdot t_s$$

where QP is the shunt ratio (ratio of oxymetrically determined shunt flow and the pulmonary blood flow), Q_p is the pulmonary flow, t_c is the average cycle time determined from ECG taken during the examination period and t_s is the average duration of the systole.

Figure 8 demonstrates the normalized oxymetrically determined flow through the ventricular septal defect as a function of the ratio $MAIS/V_{max}$. It can be recognized that between oxymetrically determined flow through the septal defect and the ratio $MAIS/V_{max}$ a linear relationship exists ($y = 0.02x + 0.001$; $r = 0.93$).

In Fig. 9 the ratio $MAIS/V_{max}$ is plotted as a function of L-R shunt expressed as % of systemic flow. As can be seen also in this case a linear relationship ($y = 0.02x - 0.08$; $r = 0.93$) between these two parameters is observed. In this figure the scatter of the data is indicated as well. The standard deviation of the grouped data on the y-axis is about ± 18%. On the x-axis the corresponding value was about ± 25%.

The method was also applied to the quantitative evaluation of atrial septal defect and for the determination of regurgitation volume in mitral valve insufficiency.

Fig. 4. Color Doppler echocardiography of 6-mth-old patient A.Chr. with ventricular septal defect; parasternal long-axis view demonstrates a perimembraneous VSD. Maximal area of the imaged shunt was 2.3 cm^2/m^2 BS. Maximal velocity was 4.4 m/s. Transducer frequency 3.5 MHz; repetition rate 6 kHz (see opposite page, top).

Fig. 5. Influence of different views. Patient J.A.; 6-mth-old patient with perimembraneous VSD L-R shunt 25% of Q_S. MAIS 0.65 cm^2/m^2 BS (short axis view [upper left]); MAIS 0.70 cm^2/m^2 BS (long axis view [upper right]); MAIS 0.85 cm^2/m^2 BS (four chamber view [lower left]); V_{max} (CW): 4 m/s Transducer frequency 3.5 MHz; repetition rate 6 kHz (see opposite page, bottom).

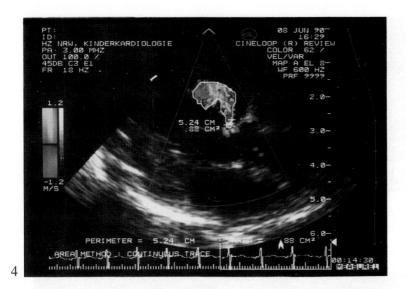

4

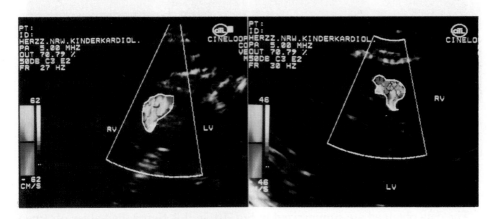

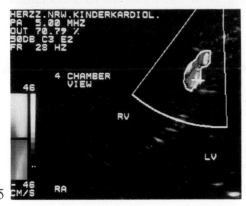

5

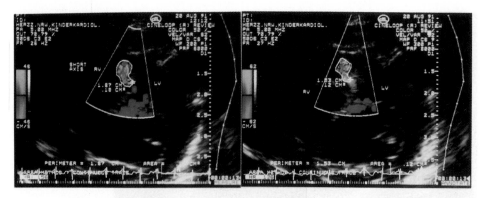

Fig. 6. Influence of different repetition rates. Patient T.F., 6-mth-old infant with perimembraneous VSD L-R shunt 25% of Q_S. MAIS 0.18 cm^2 (repetition frequency 6 kHz [left]; MAIS 0.60 cm^2/m^2 (repetition frequency 8 kHz [right]; V_{max} (CW): 4 m/s; transducer frequency 3.5 MHz.

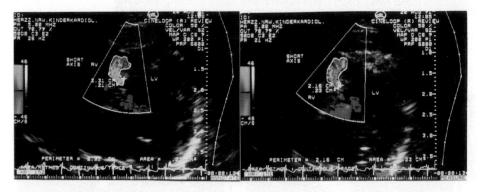

Fig. 7. Angular dependency. Patient R.S., 6-mth-old infant with perimembraneous VSD. L-R shunt 35% of Q_S. Short axis view MAIS 1.05 cm^2/m^2 (optimum beam angle [left]); MAIS 1.15 cm^2/m^2 (jet direction plus 15° [right]). Transducer frequency 3.5 MHz; repetition rate 6 kHz.

The data obtained are summarized in Fig. 10. In this figure the values obtained by noninvasive quantitative determination of left to right shunts in VSD are demonstrated as white squares and data obtained in ASDs as rhomboids. In the case of mitral valve insufficiency the data obtained echocardiographically were related to regurgitation flows determined oxymetrically. It can be seen that both VSA and MI data follow the same straight line as ASD data. This means that the proposed method might be applied even for these data.

Discussion

The primary information from color echocardiography (CDE) is the image of the jet issuing from the septal defect into right ventricular cavity. The experience

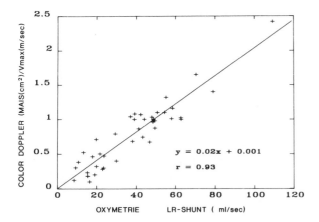

Fig. 8. Flow through the ventricular septal defect plotted as a function of the ratio MAIS/V_{max}. The flow through the septal defect corresponding to the imaged flow was calculated on the basis of following relationship: QP $\cdot$ Q_p $\cdot$ t_c/60 $\cdot$ t_s where QP is the shunt volume related to the pulmonary flow, Q_p is the pulmonary flow, t_c is the average cycle time determined from ECG taken during the examination period and t_s is the average duration of the systole.

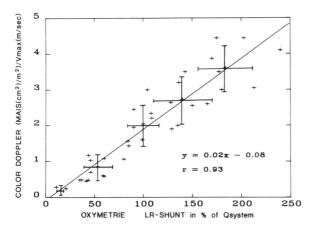

Fig. 9. The ratio of maximal area of imaged shunt (MAIS) and maximal velocity (V_{max}) plotted as a function of oxymetrically determined left to right shunt in ventricular septal defect expressed as a % of systemic flow. Both parameters were normalized to 1 m^2 of body surface. The lines plotted in represent the mean values and standard deviations of the grouped data.

with CDE obtained so far suggest that the dimension of the maximal area of the imaged shunt (MAIS) changes with the dimensions of the septal defect. Based on this observation we developed a method which permits the quantitative non-invasive determination of the shunt volume (SV) by the use of color Doppler echocardiography.

In order to explain the principles of our quantitative assessment of the shunt volume using the color image of the jet, we first considered a simple hydro-

EMPIRIC RELATIONS

Comparison of MAIS and all oxymetrically and echocardiographically determined shunt or regurgitation volume

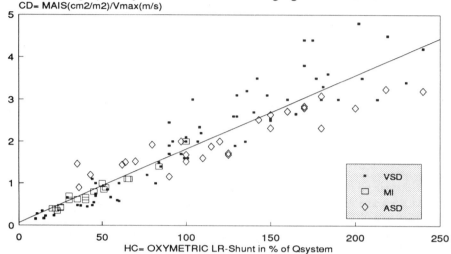

Fig. 10. In the already known regression function of oxymetrically determined left to right shunts in VSD the data of ASD and mitral valve insufficiency are compared.

dynamic system in which a jet of the fluid is expanding from an opening in the wall in a stationary medium. As demonstrated by Landau and Lifschitz [1] and Prandtl [2] in such a case the jet has the form of a cone. The opening angle of this cone was found to be fairly constant [1,2]. Based on the volume of the cone the maximal area of the cross-section in the long axis can be determined analytically. This area corresponds to the MAIS.

Since due to the suction effects [1,2] the amount of fluid in the jet is increasing from cross-section to cross-section it was not possible to analyse the properties of the jet on the basis of the mass conservation law. The physical measurements demonstrated [1,2], however, that the flow in the jet obeys the momentum flux conservation law. The momentum is given by the product of the mass of the fluid in the cone and the flow velocity. Therefore, the momentum flux conservation law was applied to solution of our problem; in a similar way the energy conservation law was used for calculation of the pressure gradients from the Doppler data.

The results of these analyses demonstrated that not the maximal area of the imaged shunt itself but the ratio of the maximal area of the imaged shunt and the maximal velocity in the septal defect (V_{max}) represents a parameter which reflects the flow in the shunt. This surprising conclusion becomes evident, however, if we recall that the MAIS at a constant flow is strongly dependent on the velocity. In the ratio between MAIS and V_{max}, the MAIS becomes normalized to a common maximal velocity and we obtain a parameter which depends only on flow.

In fact in vitro measurements [3] under ideal conditions demonstrated the linear relationship between the ratio $MAIS/V_{max}$ and the flow and definitely confirmed our conclusions.

Since the conditions met by the jet expansion in the moving right ventricle deviate significantly from those in an experimental system, the question arose how far the conclusions drawn from our analyses are applicable to results obtained in in vivo studies with color Doppler. In order to answer this question we examined a group of patients simultaneously by color Doppler echocardiography and heart catheterization.

The data obtained in patients with ASD (see Fig. 8) demonstrated that also under in vivo conditions the ratio $MAIS/V_{max}$ normalized to heart rate is linearly correlated to the actual flow through the septal defect.

At first glance one would expect that one of the possible objections to this methodology might relate to the fact that much of the shunted blood into the right ventricle does not remain in a static position and frequently and rapidly moves through the right ventricle into the pulmonary artery, i.e. at any one static moment during the systolic portion of the cardiac cycle one may determine the variable amont of shunted volume. That this conclusion is not valid becomes evident if it is considered that the echocardiographic color flow imaging does not register the fate of the single particle but provides information about the distribution of velocities in the jet. In our study we used a frame rate of 15/s. With the average heart rate of 120/min this means that there were 2 heart revolutions in 1 second and the heart revolution was resolved in 7–8 frames. Consequently the systole was registered in 2–3 frames. By detection of MAIS in ECG gated images the MAIS reflects the average distribution of the velocities in the jet during the systole, i.e. it represents the average shunt flow during the systole and not the amount of shunted volume at any one static moment during the systolic portion of the cardiac cycle. In this connection it has, however, to be pointed out that by our method the acceleration and deceleration phase of the jet development are ignored. This is probably one of the reasons for the observed scatter of the data.

After relating ECD data to actual transseptal flow we determined whether the ratio $MAIS/V_{max}$ can be related to some parameter usually used in cardiac diagnostics as well.

Since the systemic cardiac index is a parameter underlying central nervous regulation it remains in a narrow range not only with normals but also in most patients with septal defect. Therefore, it can be expected that parameters such as L-R shunt expressed as % of systemic flow will closely correlate with the shunt flow and thus with the ratio $MAIS/V_{max}$. In fact, as can be seen in Fig. 9, a close correlation between these two parameters is observed. In this figure the scatter of the data is indicated as well. The standard deviation of the data on the y-axis is about $\pm$ 18%. In the x-axis the corresponding value was about $\pm$ 25%.

These data seem to validate the conclusions of our theory and indicate that

CDE might provide a powerful tool for non-invasive quantitative determination of SV or regurgitation volume if the method described above is integrated in the configuration of the system.

Where are the limits for the application of this method in the clinical routine? In this respect two main sources of experimental error in the determination of MAIS have to be discussed.

The initial and most obvious error occurs if the MAIS is determined solely in one plane (Fig. 5). According to our experience the determinations have to be performed in long-axis, short-axis and four-chamber views. Otherwise the scatter of the data exceeds 20%. The repeated planimetric determinations of the MAIS also lead to reduction in the resulting error.

As can be seen in Fig. 6, a further source of errors might be the repetition frequency. Due to (1) normalization of the velocities to the Nyquist limit and (2) the fact that by determination of MAIS the eye always selects the same color (i.e. the same fraction of the Nyquist velocity) as the border of the imaged shunt, the MAIS is dependent on the repetition rate used. Thus the use of different repetition rates may lead to errors of up to 40%.

In contrast, the variations of the beam angle lead, surprisingly, only to small deviations in MAIS determinations.

These data indicate that the examination conditions should be normalized. In our protocol we require moreover that the patient is immobile. This can be achieved by sedation. Since, as demonstrated above, MAIS, V_{max}, shunt volume and systemic volume are heart-rate-dependent values, we require for evaluation of these parameters that the measurements are carried out at comparable heart rates. If this is not possible we carry out a heart rate correction using eq. (10). On the other hand the ratio of the MAIS to velocity as well as the shunt volume expressed as % of systemic volume are autocorrelative values, in which the effects of heart rate are eliminated. Therefore, for evaluation of these parameters no heart rate correction is necessary.

The method presented was developed for the case of a jet issuing to the right ventricle. But it can be applied to all single directed shunts imagable by the color Doppler echocardiography. So far it is not clear if this method is also applicable to patients with cross shunts. This question is the subject of our future studies.

The data presented in this study suggest that color Doppler echocardiography might in future provide a powerful tool for non-invasive quantitative determination of LR shunt of VSD/ASD and regurgitation volumes in MI.

References

1. Landau LD, Lifschitz EM (1971) Lehrbuch der theorerischen Physik IV, Hydrodynamik. Berlin: Akademie Verlag, 148–154.
2. Sass F, Bouche Ch, Leitner A (1970) Eigenschaften des freien Strahls. In: DUBBEL Taschenbuch für den Maschinenbau 13. Auflage, Erster Band. Berlin: Springer-Verlag, 320–321.

3. Sugawara M, Seo Y, Hongo H (1990) Fluid dynamics of free jets: quantification of regurgitations, shunts, and stenosed flows. In: M Sugawara, F Kajiya, A Kitabatake and H Matsuo, eds. Blood Flow in the Heart and Large Vessels. Tokyo: Springer Verlag, 173–177.
4. Wranne B, Ask P, Loyd D (1986) Quantification of heart valve regurgitation by jet intrusion. In: MP Spencer, ed. Cardiac Doppler Diagnosis, Vol. II. Dordrecht: Martinus Nijhoff, 133–140.

131

Three-dimensional shaded surface reconstructions from intravascular ultrasound B-mode images (IVUS) in vitro

R. Hammentgen[1], S. El-Gammal[2], M. Meine[1], J. Vogt[1], K.P. Mellwig[1], D. Faßbender[1], H. Schmidt[1] and U. Gleichmann[1]

[1]Kardiologische Klinik, Herzzentrum NRW, Ruhr-Universität, Georgstrasse 11, W-4970 Bad Oeynhausen, F.R.G. and [2]Dermatologische Klinik, Ruhr-Universität, Gudrunstrasse 56, W-4630 Bochum, F.R.G.

Introduction

Diagnostical ultrasound imaging systems in use today make two-dimensional sections of different organs available. By rotating, translating and tilting the B-scan applicator, a sequence of ultrasound images is available which is eventually processed and synthetically reassembled by the brain of an experienced examiner to give him a spacial understanding of structure interaction.

This in-vitro study intends to prove that the combination of parallel B-scan sections in sequence obtained from intravascular ultrasound (IVUS) with the program ANAT3D [1,3] allows one to objectify and to document the three-dimensional topographic information from ultrasound images.

In principle, two different reconstruction procedures are conceivable [3], voxel reconstructions and boundary surface reconstructions. Voxel reconstructions use volume elements to describe the total image stack. Methods like CT and NMR imaging showing few artifacts have been used successfully for voxel reconstructions. Up to now, 3D reconstructions of ultrasound images have exhibited multiple artifacts due to signal attenuation and reflection phenomena. Therefore 3D voxel reconstructions were less suited for ultrasound. This study demonstrates that boundary surface reconstructions eliminate these artifacts.

Materials

We used a CVIS-ultrasound-imaging system with several 20 (30) MHz two-dimensional imaging catheters [3]. In-vitro preparations of normal and pathological blood vessels were filled with saline solution and mounted into a fixation device (Fig. 1). The catheter was moved while registering the distance marks and storing the ultrasound images with a video recorder. Fig. 2 exhibits an IVUS-B-scan section of the right common iliac artery.

Methods

The program ANAT3D requires parallel sections in sequence [1]. The contours of all structures of interest are entered into the computer section by section using a video processing unit and a pointing device to draw the polygonal outline of the structures. After calibration all objects are reconstructed in their true dimensions, allowing exact volume and surface calculations. By automatically choosing the appropriate magnification according to the structures selected, the objects are then transformed into an integer space. This procedure makes it easy to study very large and/or very small objects with an optimal resolution. To analyse structure interaction, a set of different presentation modes is available for every structure (surface reconstruction, wire model, line model, point cloud). By combining these different presentation modes, structures within structures are easily visualized. On the other hand, in-depth shading and/or surface shading by a virtual point light source improves picture interpretation considerably.

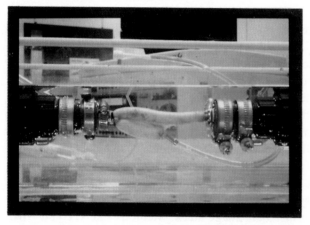

Fig. 1. Device to study blood vessels in vitro. Note the vessel mounted between two floodgates.

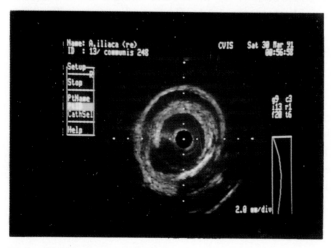

Fig. 2. 20 MHz intravascular B-scan image of the right common iliac artery. Different layers of the vessel wall can be recognized.

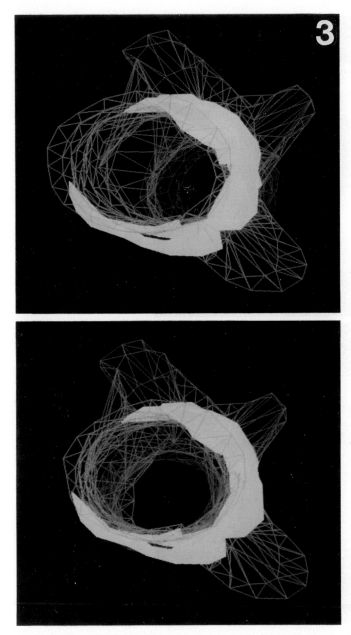

Fig. 3. Stereoscopic 3D reconstruction of the right subclavian artery (red, wire-frame mode) of a 68-yr-old man (5F, 30 MHz CVIS catheter). The internal mammary artery points downwards and the thyrocervical trunk points upwards. 37 sections, total length 6.2 cm. Note the arteriosclerotic plaque (yellow, surface-mode).

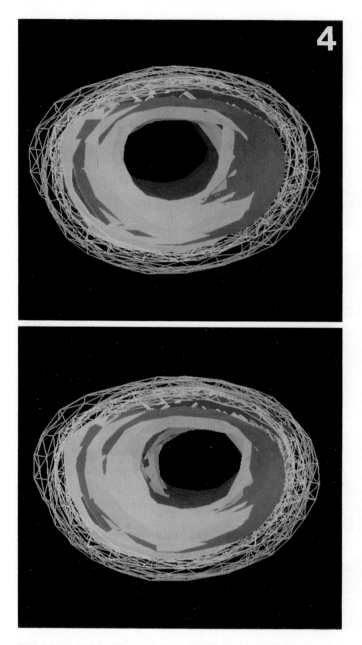

Fig. 4. Stereoscopic 3D reconstruction of the left external iliac artery (red: inner vessel wall; green: outer vessel wall) of a 70-yr-old man (8F, 20 MHz CVIS catheter). Note the extensive arteriosclerotic plaques (yellow). 34 sections, total length 6.8 cm.

By tilting the objects 2–4 degrees, stereoscopic image pairs can be obtained, comparable to the wax-plate reconstructions in the past. Red/green techniques allow true 3D models in black-and-white, while polaroscopic techniques enable true colour 3D models. The stereoscopic image pairs can be printed as hard copies (prismatic glasses) or can be projected with a stereoprojector (polaroscopic glasses).

Results

By using an intravascular imaging-catheter we were able to plausibly reconstruct central arteries and veins. Existing plaques were easily differentiated and could be measured in their obstruction volume (within the 3D models). In the region of plaques (yellow structure in Figs. 3 and 4), the thickness of the neighbouring media (violet) was reduced. Figs. 3 and 4 are stereo pairs which can be visualized with prismatic glasses (Balzers Union, Lichtenstein).

Note the bifurcation of the subclavian artery in Fig. 3 (red wire-frame) with the internal mammary artery facing downwards and the thyrocervical trunk facing upwards. Figure 4 exhibits an arteriosclerotic left external iliac artery.

Discussion

The above-mentioned results show that a successful 3D reconstruction from serial ultrasound B-scan sections using intravascular two-dimensional imaging catheters is possible. In this reported experimental setup, the precise orientation and determination of the B-scan sections was easy. However, in vivo, a precise and reproducible geometric orientation of the ultrasonic transducer is much more difficult. When these mechanical problems are solved, it is expected that the arteriosclerotic plaque volume and other surface/volume parameters can be determined, providing a quantitative follow-up of cardiovascular pathology. Using transesophageal echocardiographic probes, we could already demonstrate the feasibility of 3D reconstructions of the aorta in vivo [2].

Furthermore, the subjective intraindividual perception and conceptualization of spatial relationships between different structure components can now be objectified and documented. Using stereoscopic techniques even 3D imaging is possible.

Thus, the geometric accuracy of the 3D models using boundary reconstruction procedures are only limited by the precision of the mechanical procedure during image acquisition.

References

1. El-Gammal S, Altmeyer P, Hinrichsen K (1989) ANAT3D: Shaded three-dimensional surface reconstructions from serial sections. Acta Stereol Suppl 8/2: 543–550.

2. Hammentgen R, El-Gammal S, Hausmann M, Bergbauer M, Ricken D (1990) Three-dimensional surface reconstructions of cardiac and paracardiac structures. International Symposium on Echocardiography, Mainz, Kongressband B 33.
3. Hammentgen R (1991) Transösophageale Echocardiographie monoplan/biplan. Atlas und Lehrbuch. Berlin: Springer-Verlag.

Surgical reconstruction of cardiac valves

Carlos M.G. Duran

Department of Cardiovascular Diseases, King Faisal Specialist Hospital and Research Center, P.O. Box 3354, Riyadh 1211, Saudi Arabia

Mitral valve repair

The mitral valve, probably because of its frequent involvement and long-standing exposure to the surgeon since the early days of open mitral commissurotomy, is the valve most often repaired. In fact, it has reached such a level of universal acceptance that it is now customary to state that valve replacement is only performed when repair was not possible. However, the wide disparity in rates of repair versus replacement in the different centers, and even within the same unit, shows that there is a lack of objective parameters indicating the appropriateness of repair or replacement.

Indications
A repaired valve does not require anticoagulation as such; therefore the age, sex, geographic location and sociocultural level of the patient are important factors to bear in mind. In some cases these factors will stretch the indications towards repair even in the presence of very deteriorated valves where a perfect result is unlikely. This is very relevant in young patients and particularly in fertile women where anticoagulation represents a very serious problem. In other cases such as elderly patients where a bioprosthetic replacement is known to perform satisfactorily, a difficult repair might not be indicated.

The whole field of reconstructive surgery pivots on the pathology of the valve. A preoperative transthoracic and intraoperative transesophageal echocardiographic study is essential to carefully analyse the whole mitral apparatus. A systemic approach must be used determining the annulus size, leaflet thickness and mobility, commissural fusion, presence and localization of calcific nodules, areas of prolapse and billowing, direction of the regurgitant jets, thickness and length of chords and papillary muscles.

Surgical techniques
The specific reconstruction manoeuvres are well known and have been widely published [6,10]. Some of them can be considered perfectly standardized and therefore easy and safe to perform. Quadrangular resection of the flail portion of the posterior leaflet, often present in degenerative disease, is one of them. Anterior leaflet resection, on the other hand, is seldom performed. Chordal shortening by either splitting the papillary muscle head and sliding it downwards,

or by looping the elongated chord and placating it into the papillary muscle, is also a standard technique [3]. Chord replacement with a Goretex suture is still too recent a development to class it as established [4]. Chordal transfer from the posterior to the anterior leaflet is an easy and well-established procedure [5]. Cusp extension with pericardium, although promising, needs a longer follow-up before it has wide acceptance [6,7]. All these manoeuvres must be followed by a ring annuloplasty. Two types of prosthetic ring are currently used: the Carpentier rigid ring [8] and the Duran flexible ring [9]. The difference between the two models is that the rigid Carpentier ring is designed to the systolic shape of the mitral annulus whilst the Duran ring, because of its flexibility, follows the normal changes in the shape of the annulus during the cardiac cycle. Recent experimental work by Van Rijk-Zwiker et al. [10] has shown that the flexible ring during systole acquires the systolic shape of the mitral and therefore is similar to a Carpentier ring, while during diastole it becomes more circular and therefore less stenotic. A superior left ventricular function after a flexible ring implantation has also been shown, both experimentally [10] and clinically [11]. Furthermore, a problem with systolic anterior motion secondary to the placement of a rigid ring has been repeatedly described in the literature, while so far absent after the use of a flexible ring [12,13]. From a surgical point of view, a flexible ring reduces the tension of the sutures, decreasing the likelihood of ring dehiscence.

Results

Generally, the clinical results of mitral valve repair are superior to those of mitral valve replacement. A recent review by David [14] of the literature showed a compounded hospital mortality for mitral stenosis of 0.9% for repair versus 7.3% for replacement, and in mitral regurgitation 3.4% for repair versus 10.6% for replacement. This significant difference is probably due to the better left ventricular function following mitral repair where the annulo-ventricular continuity is preserved [15]. It remains to be seen whether this difference is maintained when the results of replacement with conservation of the chordal attachments become available.

The incidence of thromboembolism, hemorrhagic complications and infective endocarditis is definitely lower after mitral valve repair than after replacement [16]. The actuarial survival after mitral valve repair is greater than after valve replacement [17]. All these figures, however, do not take into account that these are not randomized studies and therefore the different patient populations might be biased towards performing repairs in less complicated patients.

Aortic valve repair

Faced with a young population where anticoagulation represents a very serious problem and who frequently suffer from concomitant mitral lesions which have been successfully repaired, we adopted a similar conservative attitude for the aortic valve. After nearly 20 years of this approach, we can now consider that in selected patients aortic repair can be safely undertaken.

Surgical techniques

The same general principles for repair of the mitral valve apply to the aortic valve. The lesions must be carefully analysed and treated individually. Intraoperative echocardiography is mandatory.

The conservative surgical techniques applied fall into two distinct categories: those patients judged to have enough valvular tissue undergo a variety of techniques directed towards achieving competence without the use of any extra valvular tissue [18]. These techniques, grouped under the heading of 'repair', should be taken as a whole, as usually each of them only achieves partial improvement and requires reinforcement by others (Fig. 1). A review of the long-term results obtained from a group of 50 patients who underwent an operation with these techniques from 1974 showed a 13-year actuarial survival of 86% and only 4 reoperations due to severe aortic dysfunction [19]. These techniques include: (a) commissurotomy, always performed in the presence of even minimal fusion in order to maximize cusp mobility; (b) unrolling of the free edge of each leaflet, which increases the area by a few millimeters; (c) annuloplasty by means of the placement of a pledgeted 'U' stitch at the base of each commissure, which by placating the aortic wall reduces its total circumference; (d) in those cases with prolapse, the resuspension of the cusp free edge is also performed following the technique described by Trusler [20]; and finally (e) in some cases an enhance-

Aortic Valve Repair - Reduced Cusp Mobility

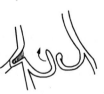
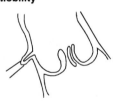

Commissurotomy   Free Edge Unrolling   Cusp Shaving

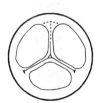
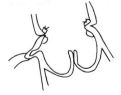
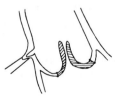

Ca^{++} Excision   Ridge Enhancement   Cusp Extension

Fig. 1. Aortic valve repair techniques. (Reproduced with permission from Ann Thorac Surg 1991; 52: 447–454.)

ment of the supraaortic ridge is induced in order to improve the valve hemo-dynamics [21].

In the presence of very severe cusp retraction, these manoeuvres cannot be used and extension of all three cusps is performed with a single strip of fashioned glutaraldehyde-treated pericardium. Two main questions must be addressed when considering the use of this approach. The first is the need for a standard surgical technique that ensures a correct, reproducible and safe result in terms of immediate competence. The second is the long-term durability of the selected material. We recently reviewed our experience in a group of 45 patients who had a cusp extension with pericardium. There was no hospital mortality with a maximum follow-up of 3 years. There were no late deaths or embolic events although none was anticoagulated. The mean preoperative degree of regurgitation was 3.24 ± 0.1 (grades 0–4+). The mean intraoperative regurgitation post-repair was 0.59 ± 0.5, which was maintained throughout the follow-up period. There were two reoperations in this group of patients, but both were due to dysfunction of the simultaneously performed mitral repair. In both of them the aortic valve was inspected, revealing pliable pericardium at 4 and 8 mth post-surgery. This technique can now be considered standardized and reproducible.

The absence of a rigid stent when used in cusp extension, however, not only reduces the transvalvular gradient, especially important in very young patients, but also reduces the tissue stress, hopefully increasing its durability. Even in the event of failure, the excision of the calcified pericardium should be easy, given that the patient's leaflet remnants have been preserved. The recent report by Chachques et al. [22] of the biological advantages of glutaraldehyde-treated autologous pericardium encouraged us to use it in the last 20 cases, with excellent results to date.

Indications for aortic valve repair

As in the case of mitral valve repair, the indications for aortic valve repair depend primarily on the lesions encountered. Calcified valves are beyond repair given that the different attempts at decalcification have been shown to be very short-lived. However, isolated calcific nodules, particularly those often found at the level of one fused commissure, can be shaven from the inflow aspect of the leaflets after commisurotomy. Very thick and rigid valves are also beyond the possibility of present-day reconstruction. Those valves with minimal or moderate fibrosis of the leaflet base are good candidates for repair. In many young rheumatic patients the only cause of regurgitation is the presence of rolled-in, thick, free edges that can be unrolled followed by annuloplasty. If the degree of cusp retraction is too important, cusp extension is indicated. In these cases, however, because the long-term durability of the glutaraldehyde-treated autologous pericardium is still unknown, we reserve this technique for young patients where anticoagulation is a problem.

Tricuspid valve repair

The tricuspid valve, because less often affected, has followed the development in the surgery of the other valves and in particular the mitral valve. At present, stenosis is treated by open commissurotomy [23] and regurgitant lesions by annuloplasty. The technique described by Kay et al. [24], which consisted of transformation of the tricuspid orifice into a bicuspid valve by plication of the posterior leaflet area, has been practically abandoned because the correction does not withstand the test of time. The semicircular annuloplasty proposed by Cabrol [25] and DeVega [26] uses a double continuous suture that reduced the annulus at the level of the anterior and posterior leaflets without interfering with the base of the septal leaflet, which is normally not dilated. A different approach was described by Carpentier et al. in 1971 [8] in which they used a preshaped rigid prosthetic ring of different sizes, which was sutured to the tricuspid annulus and reduced it selectively. We [9] have described a flexible ring which follows the same principle. However, its flexibility adapts better to the continuous changes in the shape and size of the normal tricuspid orifice. At least theoretically, it would be less prone to dehiscence and to induce stenosis because of its ability to become more circular during diastole.

Indications

The vast majority of the tricuspid valve lesions can be repaired. The problem rather lies in diagnosing its presence, degree of regurgitation and whether it is organic or functional. Two-dimensional colour Doppler echocardiography has become a very reliable instrument, provided the tricuspid valve is systematically and carefully analysed.

Our present-day indications for tricuspid valve repair are: (1) All organic lesions should undergo a commissurotomy, followed by a flexible ring annulo-plasty. Ignoring the lesion on the basis of the small gradient present before surgery is dangerous as it is likely to become significant due to the postoperative increase in cardiac output, secondary to the repair of the left sided lesions [27]. (2) Functional regurgitation should be treated by an annuloplasty unless very mild. Those patients with a moderate regurgitation and low pulmonary (arteriolar) resistance should undergo a simple DeVega-type annuloplasty. In these cases it can be expected that the right ventricular failure will improve after the reduction in afterload following the mitral repair. The annuloplasty is directed towards an improved postoperative period.

The patients with a severe regurgitation should undergo a ring annuloplasty. It is felt that the degree of annular dilatation would impose too much strain on a DeVega suture.

Results

Because of the characteristics of the tricuspid valve the results of its repair are very difficult to analyse objectively. The hospital mortality varies between 4 and

31% [28]. In a series of 359 patients who underwent tricuspid repair between 1974 and 1979 at our Institution, the hospital mortality was 8.4% [27]. More recently in a series of 172 patients who had a tricuspid repair performed between 1988 and 1991, the hospital mortality was 4%. This disparity in mortality rates reported in the literature is not primarily due to the different types of repair, but rather to the preoperative condition of the patient.

We have also shown that the postoperative function and more importantly the cardiac output of the patients are directly related to the results of the surgery on the left-sided lesions and not with the hemodynamic results of the tricuspid surgery [27]. Postoperative hemodynamic Doppler studies have shown residual transvalvular gradients in a significant number of patients after annuloplasty. Residual insufficiency was also frequent, although clearly related to the presence of postoperative mitral dysfunction. In spite of these problems, tricuspid valve repair is universally accepted as far superior to tricuspid replacement, which carries a much higher risk of endocarditis or thrombosis.

The rate of tricuspid repair versus replacement is the highest among the cardiac valves. In our reported series, out of 368 patients operated for tricuspid disease, where 50% had organic disease, only 9 (2.4%) had a replacement [27]. It can be concluded that, although not yet perfect, repair has become the procedure of choice in tricuspid valve surgery.

References

1. Carpentier A (1984) Valve reconstruction in predominant mitral valve incompetence. In: C Duran, WW Angell, AD Johnson and JJ Oury, eds. Recent Progress in Mitral Valve Disease. London: Butterworths, 265-274.
2. Duran CMG (1984) Mitral reconstruction in predominant mitral stenosis. In: CG Duran, WW Angell, AD Johnson and JH Oury, eds. Recent Progress in Mitral Valve Disease. London: Butterworths, 255-264.
3. Duran CMG (1989) Surgical management of elongated chordae of the mitral valve. J Cardiac Surg 4: 253-260.
4. David TE (1989) Replacement of chordae tendinea with expanded polytetrafluoroethylene sutures. J Cardiac Surg 4: 286-290.
5. Duran CG (1986) Repair of anterior mitral leaflet chordal rupture or elongation (the flip-over technique). J Cardiac Surg 1: 161-166.
6. Gallo JI, Duran CMG (1980) Uso clinico del pericardio heterologo tratado con glutaraldehido para la ampliacion del velo valvular mitral. Rev Cir Esp 34: 63-68.
7. Chauvaud SM, Chachques JM, Mihaileanu S, et al. (1990) Valvular extension with autologous pericardium preserved with glutaraldehyde. Results in mitral valve repair (Abstract). Am Ass Thorac Surg Meeting, May 1990.
8. Carpentier A, Deloche A, Dauptain J, et al. (1971) A new reconstructive operation for correction of mitral and tricuspid insufficiency. J Thorac Cardiovasc Surg 61: 1-13.
9. Duran CMG, Ubago JL (1976) Clinical and hemodynamic performance of a totally flexible prosthetic ring for atrioventricular valve reconstruction. Ann Thorac Surg 22: 458-463.
10. Van Rijk-Zwikker GL, Mast F, Schipperheyn JJ, et al. (1990) Comparison of rigid and flexible rings for annuloplasty of the porcine mitral valve. Circulation 82(Suppl IV): 58-64.

11. David TE, Komeda M, Pollick C, et al. (1989) Mitral valve annuloplasty. The effect of the type on left ventricular function. Ann Thorac Surg 47: 524–527.
12. Kreindel MS, Schiavone WA, Lever HM, et al. (1986) Systolic anterior motion of the mitral valve after Carpentier's ring valvuloplasty for mitral valve prolapse. Am J Cardiol 57: 408–412.
13. Grossi EA, Galloway AC, Colvin SB, et al. (1991) Experience with 28 cases of systolic anterior motion after Carpentier mitral valve reconstruction (Abstract). Am Assoc Thoracic Meeting, May 1991.
14. David TE (1990) A rational approach to the surgical treatment of mitral valve disease. In: RB Karp, ed. Advances in Cardiac Surgery. Chicago: Mosby Year Book, Vol 2, 63–84.
15. David TE, Burns RJ, Bacchus CM, et al. (1984) Mitral valve replacement for mitral regurgitation with and without preservation of chordae tendinea. J Thorac Cardiovasc Surg 88: 718–725.
16. Perier P, Deloche A, Chauvaud S, et al. (1984) Comparative evaluation of mitral valve repair and replacement with Starr, Bjork and porcine valve prostheses. Circulation 70(Suppl I): 187–192.
17. Galloway AC, Colvin SB, Baumann FG, et al. (1988) Current concepts in mitral valve reconstruction for mitral insufficiency. Circulation 78: 1087–1098.
18. Duran CMG (1988) Reconstructive techniques for rheumatic aortic valve disease. J Cardiac Surg 3: 23–28.
19. Duran CMG, Alonso J, Gaite L, et al. (1988) Long term results of conservative repair of the rheumatic aortic valve insufficiency. Eur J Cardio-Thorac Surg 2: 217–223.
20. Trusler GA, Moes CA, Kidd BS (1973) Repair of ventricular septal defect with aortic insufficiency. J Thorac Cardiovasc Surg 66: 394–403.
21. Duran CMG, Balasundaram S, Bianchi S, et al. (1990) Hemodynamic effect of supraaortic ridge enhancement on the closure mechanism of the aortic valve and its implication in aortic valve repair. Thorac Cardiovasc Surgeon 38: 6–10.
22. Chachques JC, Vasseur B, Perrier P, et al. (1988) A rapid method to stabilize biological materials for cardiovascular surgery. Ann New York Acad Sc 529: 184–186.
23. Revuelta JM, Garcia R, Duran CMG (1985) Tricuspid commissurotomy. Ann Thorac Surg 39: 489–491.
24. Kay JH, Maselli-Campagna G, Tsuji KK (1965) Surgical treatment of tricuspid insufficiency. Ann Surg 162: 53–58.
25. Cabrol C (1972) Annuloplastie valvulaire. Un nouveau procede. Nouv Pres Med 1: 1366.
26. DeVega N (1972) La Anuloplastia selectiva, regulable y permanente. Unea tecnica original para el tratamiento de la insuficiencia tricuspide. Rev Esp Cardiol 25: 555–560.
27. Duran CMG, Pomar JL, Colman T, et al. (1980) Is tricuspid valve repair necessary? J Thorac Cardiovasc Surg 80: 849–860.
28. De Paulis R, Bobbio M, Ottino G, et al. (1990) The DeVega tricuspid annuloplasty. Preoperative mortality and long term follow-up. J Cardiovasc Surg 31: 512–517.

Stentless porcine bioprosthesis valve replacement

William W. Angell, Dennis F. Pupello, Luis N. Bessone and Stephen P. Hiro

Joseph's Heart Institute, Tampa, FL, U.S.A.

Use of biological valves began in 1956 when Heimbecker and Murray used fresh unsupported homograft tissue sewn directly into the descending thoracic aorta with a double row of sutures [1]. In 1958, Duran and Gunning proved experimentally that fresh transplanted homograft valves could be made competent in the subcoronary position when secured with a single row of running sutures [2]. With the advent of cardiopulmonary bypass these two principles were later applied clinically by Ross and Barratt-Boyes in 1961 [3,4]. Homografts have subsequently been prepared in a variety of ways and used in several thousand cases as unstented orthotopic aortic valve replacements secured with two suture lines [5].

The first series of xenograft valves in patients was reported by O'Brien in 1966 in Brisbane, Australia. He used a valve composed of three porcine valve non-coronary leaflets packed with cotton wool and soaked in a weak formaldehyde solution [6]. The resultant tanned graft was secured with a single running suture in 127 patients. Early clinical results were excellent. The reported hospital mortality for the series was 4.0%. Implanted valves sounded normal by auscultation and none required early reoperation for incompetence. Concomitantly at Stanford University in California, Angell and Buch implanted whole porcine valves secured to a ridged metal stent and packed with cotton wool and soaked in a similar pH-controlled 1% formalin solution [7]. The hospital mortality for this group of patients was also low at 5.0%. Valves implanted were found to be competent without early failure.

The formalin tissue in both series deteriorated rapidly, lasting only 2.3 yr on average in the California stented valves and 5.5 yr in the Australian experience with unstented composite grafts (Fig. 1). These two experiences suggest that the single suture line was sufficient for implantation of the unstented valves because of the natural tough fibrous tissue present at the base of the non-coronary leaflet. It also suggests that the composite unstented valve was more durable than the similarly tanned but stented valve. Subsequent rapid acceptance of the commercial stent-mounted glutaraldehyde-treated porcine valve has resulted in an excellent clinical experience well documented from many major centers over the ensuing 20 yr. An unfortunate outcome of this success was that it precluded further clinical trials to test the comparison of stented versus unstented glutaraldehyde-treated porcine tissue valves.

From 1968 to 1975, just prior to the original experiences with glutaraldehyde porcine xenografts, Angell and Shumway started a series comparing stented and unstented fresh antibiotic sterilized homografts in 450 patients. These tissue valves functioned well. Over the 20-yr follow-up it became clear that like the prior experience with formalin-fixed tissue, stent-mounted homografts were less durable than if stentless valves were sutured directly into the aortic root. Stented valves failed at 9 yr on average, while unstented grafts had a mean time to structural deterioration of 14 yr (Fig. 2).

Calcific degeneration appears to be the only identified patient-related factor which clearly affects valve durability. Not only did the stent-mounted homografts

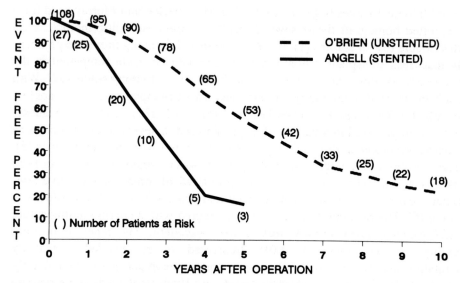

Fig. 1. Freedom from structural deterioration for stented and unstented aortic valve replacement formaldehyde treated xenografts.

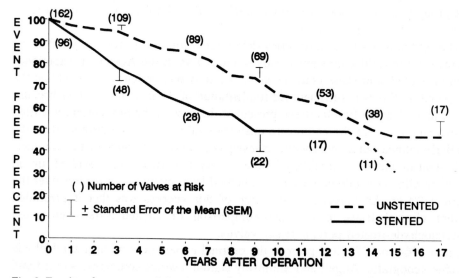

Fig. 2. Freedom from structural deterioration for stented and unstented aortic homografts.

and xenografts have the same freedom from structural deterioration but there was also a similar tendency for calcification as a failure mode of these two valve types [8]. The decreased tendency for unstented valves to calcify may in part explain their increased durability. The calcific degeneration of stented xenografts is clearly an age-related phenomenon, with grafts functioning for only a few years in children [9] and for greater than 15 yr in elderly patients [10]. Our third observation was that this age relation to structural deterioration occurred in stented but not unstented homografts.

Results from this homograft experience also raise the question as to whether or not the unstented xenograft may calcify less and thus be more durable if sewn directly to the aortic wall. In 1975, Angell implanted a small number of unstented valves using a standard homograft two suture line method, but with grafts that were glutaraldehyde-treated rather than exposed to formalin [11]. Ten years later, David, Bernard and Ross also reported on unstented and semi-stented techniques for glutaraldehyde treated xenograft valve insertion [12-14]. The rationale for using a graft with a flexible annulus, a less obstructed orifice, and elimination of stent turbulence applies to the semi-stented as well as the unstented valve. Unfortunately, these four series [10-14] are too small for the rate of structural deterioration to add to the existing body of knowledge comparing stented and unstented tissue. As a result, we are now left with insufficient data to answer the major question as to whether the use of unstented tissue valves will significantly affect structural deterioration of glutaraldehyde porcine xenografts.

In addition to permitting the valve to be used in all intracardiac positions, stents have the obvious advantage of standardizing insertion methods with great versatility and flexibility related to the recipient anatomy. Partial stents also address the issue vital to all implant surgeons as to whether a potential increase in durability compensates for the longer operative time associated with unstented valve insertion.

Stent abrasion is a well recognized in vitro observation which has not been assessed through proper studies. While presumed to be unimportant clinically it has been observed and may play a critical role in the observed difference in structural deterioration between stented and unstented valves.

Complex techniques associated with unstented valve insertion and the requisite prolonged surgical time further serve to compound the issue. It is apparent from a limited number of experiences that whole root homograft implants result in a more natural valve configuration [15]. There is also a suggestion that this lower incidence of early valve incompetence may enhance long-term durability. Thus the whole homograft root may be more durable than the standard subcoronary valve implant. These observations have influenced the attitude of experienced biological graft surgeons to consider the advisability of using unstented rather than stented tissue for aortic replacement and to employ techniques which provide for root rather than isolated valve replacement [16,17].

The antithesis of the argument for use of the whole root is the extensive experience of O'Brien with the composite fibrous non-coronary cusp valve [6].

Although based on an entirely different concept, durability of composite valves is proven. The O'Brien valve addresses the question of rapid and versatile implantation by a single running suture at the same time as applying the principles behind the use of unstented grafts. While the reported increased durability (Fig. 1) with unstented formalin valves appears real, the extension of this conclusion to glutaraldehyde-fixed valves has not been proven and will remain controversial well into the future.

Clinical experiences (Fig. 2) comparing stented with unstented grafts and the trend toward the use of unstented aortic roots for homograft valve replacement has led us to design two types of unstented xenografts. Working with O'Brien and Bravo Cardiovascular (Irvine, CA) we began the construction of composite glutaraldehyde-treated porcine xenografts. These xenografts have been modeled after the original O'Brien valve and designed for simple suture line implantation (Fig. 3). The non-coronary leaflet is excised from equal-sized porcine valves and configured into a composite by alignment of the central corpora and the upper edges of the leaflets. The coaptive surfaces are then accentuated by suturing the cut edge of the aorta between the leaflets inferiorly. This permits commissure flexibility without disturbing valve competence. The tough fibrous tissue at the base of the non-coronary leaflet ensures leaflet integrity and permits use of a single monofilament suture to secure the valve to the host annulus (Fig. 4). The valve is then carefully positioned in the supra-annular location, so that only the

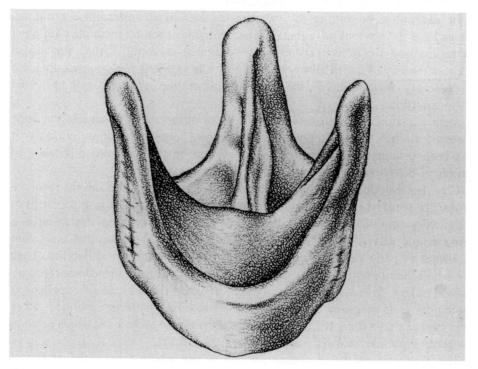

Fig. 3. O'Brien composite glutaraldehyde porcine xenograft.

leaflet itself intrudes into the aortic outflow tract, thus minimizing valve gradients even in 17–19 mm sizes. To date, there is no reported instance of dehiscence of the valve from the recipient aorta using this simple and rapid method of implantation.

Unstented porcine xenografts can also be used for total aortic root replacement or as a scalloped subcoronary graft secured with two suture lines identical to the techniques employed for homograft valve replacement. As with the O'Brien valve the long-term clinical results with these grafts remain unknown at present as they have only been employed sporadically in a limited number of cases to date. Use of the whole aortic root or two suture line technique of insertion is somewhat more complex but has the same theoretical advantages as other unstented grafts.

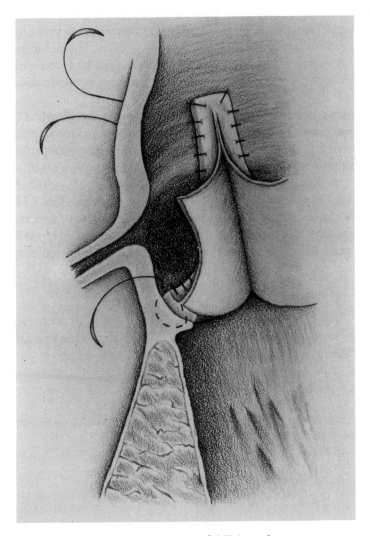

Fig. 4. Single suture line implantation of O'Brien valve.

While these grafts can be sewn directly to the recipient aortic root without the use of reinforcement material, there has been a trend toward covering of the muscular areas of the graft in order to facilitate suture placement at the time of implantation.

There exists only speculation to date as to the clinical significance of increased longevity of stented versus unstented valves. Relief of leaflet stress by flexibility of the commissure at the annulus [18], reduced turbulence around the stent, decreased tendency to calcify and less possibility of leaflet abrasion against prosthetic surfaces are four of the most common contributing mechanisms influencing structural deterioration with unstented grafts. There are clear in vitro data regarding decreased stress with flexible versus rigid commissural attachments. There has been, however, no difference observed clinically in durability with flexible versus rigid stents. Turbulent flow is known to influence calcification. The elimination of the stent may well influence this primary cause of early structural deterioration. It is further postulated that if calcification can be eliminated by the use of calcium-mitigating agents, we may well be faced with a secondary problem of leaflet abrasion previously obscured by the calcification process.

Based on these observations, the following conclusions can be drawn: (1) unstented homograft valves last longer than stented; (2) unstenting of xenografts for aortic valve replacement or root replacement is possible; and (3) partial stenting and composite non-coronary leaflet construction enhance the implantation of aortic valves.

We can further speculate from available clinical experiences that: (1) elimination of stents with xenografts may improve durability; (2) partial stents may improve durability; (3) patient factors such as age and the tendency towards calcification may be reduced by stent elimination; and (4) stent abrasion may affect long-term durability of the graft.

Acknowledgements

The authors would like to acknowledge the technical assistance provided by Dr. George Ebra and Dr. Debra Guest in the preparation of this publication.

References

1. Heimbecker RO, et al. (1962) Homograft replacement of the human mitral valve: a preliminary report. Canad Med Assoc J 86: 805–809.
2. Duran CG, Gunning AJ (1962) A method for placing a total homologous aortic valve in the subcoronary position. Lancet 2: 488–489.
3. Ross DN (1962) Homograft replacement of the aortic valve. 2: 487.
4. Barratt-Boyes BG (1964) Homograft aortic valve replacement in aortic incompetence and stenosis. Thorax 19: 131.
5. Barratt-Boyes BG (1965) A method for preparing and inserting a homograft aortic valve. Brit J Surg 52: 847–856.

6. O'Brien MF (1967) Heterograft aortic valves for human use: valve bank, techniques of measurement, and implantation. J Thorac Cardiovasc Surg 53: 392.

7. Buch WS, Kosek JC, Angell WW, Shumway NE (1970) Deterioration of formalin-treated aortic valve heterografts. J Thorac Cardiovasc Surg 60: 673-677.

8. Angell WW, Angell JD, Oury JH, et al. (1987) Long-term follow-up of viable frozen aortic homografts. J Thorac Cardiovasc Surg 93(6): 665-674.

9. Odell JA (1982) Calcification of porcine bioprostheses in children. In: LH Cohn and V Gallucci, eds. Cardiac Bioprostheses, Proceedings of the Second International Symposium. New York: Yorke Medical Books, 231-237.

10. Pupello DF, Bessone LN, Hiro SP, et al. (1991) Bioprosthetic valve durability in the elderly. Presented at the V International Symposium Cardiac Bioprosthesis, Palais Des Papes, Avignon, France, May 24-27.

11. Angell WW (1975) Unpublished data.

12. David TE, Ropchan GC, Butany JW (1988) Aortic valve replacement with stentless porcine bioprosthesis. J Cardiac Surg 3: 501-505.

13. Sievers HH, Lange PE, Bernhard A (1980) Implantation of a xenogenic stentless aortic bioprosthesis. First experience. J Thorac Cardiovasc Surg 33: 225.

14. Ross DN, Valentino R (1991) Presented at the V International Symposium Cardiac Bioprosthesis, Palais Des Papes, Avignon, France, May 24-27.

15. Yacoub MH (1987) Allograft aortic root replacement. In: AC Yankah, R Hetzer, DC Miller, et al., eds. Cardiac Valve Allografts 1962-1987. Berlin: Steinkopff Verlag Darmstadt 149-155.

16. O'Brien MF, Stafford G, Gardner M, et al. (1987) The viable cryopreserved allograft aortic valve. J Cardiac Surg 1 (Suppl): 153-167.

17. Angell WW, Pupello DF, Bessone LN, et al. (1991) Universal method for insertion of unstented aortic autografts, homografts and xenografts. Presented at the 71st Annual Meeting of the American Association of Thoracic Surgery, Washington, DC, May 6-8.

18. Reis RL, Hancock WD, Yarborough HW, et al. (1971) The flexible stent. J Thorac Cardiovasc Surg 62: 683.

Cardio-thoracic surgery. K. Minami et al. editors.

The use of aortic valve homografts: technique and results

A.J. Dziatkowiak[1], R. Pfitzner[1], J. Sadowski[1], W. Tracz[1], Z. Marek[2] and P. Podolec[1]

[1]Institute of Cardiology and [2]Department of Forensic Medicine, N. Copernicus School of Medicine, Jagiellonian University, Cracow, Poland

Introduction

Since no entirely satisfactory synthetic valve is available, the use of 'fresh', unstented, antibiotic sterilized allograft (homograft) for replacement of aortic valve, aortic root or for correction of some complex congenital malformations is emphasized by many authors [1,2,14-16]. The well-documented follow-up studies demonstrate that the results of aortic allograft implantation are comparable or better than those of mechanical valves [3-9].

Allografts are well tolerated and behave like the native valves. The further advantages are no need for anticoagulation, no thromboembolic complications, higher security in cases with severe damage because of active endocarditis, and significantly less bleeding during the aortic root replacement for aneurysms. However, degenerative changes and calcifications occur. Fortunately, in the majority of cases, they are not of clinical importance for many years [22,24].

Allografts have been used in Poland since 1974 [10-13]. In Krakow the antibiotic-sterilized, free-hand aortic valve allografts have been used since 1980. The aim of this report is to show the graft collection, storing, technique of implantation and to summarize the clinical results of 412 patients (329 males and 83 females, aged 11 to 71, mean 40 yr) in whom we inserted aortic valve homografts in subcoronary position for aortic valve replacement as a native valve or as a 'short cylinder', and for ascending aortic aneurysm replacement as a 'long cylinder'.

Material and Methods

From 1980 to July 1991 we performed 1373 aortic valve replacements, among which there were 412 aortic valve or root implantations using 'fresh', free-hand, antibiotic-sterilized homografts. The grafts were collected at the Forensic Medicine Department during the elective postmortem examination (under non-sterile condition) of previously healthy, accidentally deceased persons under 50 yr of age, not later than 48 h after death in winter and 24 h in summer time. Grafts were transferred in cold +4°C sterile saline solution to our hospital-based homograft bank. The overbounded tissue was excised and the specimen preserved in sterilizing medium at +4°C for 24 h and then transferred into the nutrient medium and stored sterile at +4°C up to 21 days. The definitive preparation and trimming was performed by the surgeon during operation after selection by size and quality. The blood group compatibility of the donor and recipient was not obligatory. More details are published elsewhere [3,4,8,9,13]. Recently we incorporated deep freezing of sterile homografts. All grafts were implanted subcoronary after removal of the affected native aortic valve.

Initially 100 homografts were implanted in place of the excised native valve using single interrupted sutures for annular anastomosis, and a running suture for the distal margin anastomosis, ommiting coronary ostia. Beforehand, the commissures were fixed and suspended by three single mattress sutures, exercising caution to prevent distortion. The last 238 homografts were sewn with a modified technique: total aortic bulb (Valsalva sinuses) with valve, as a short cuff of ascending aorta or a 'short cylinder' was inserted and sutured intra-luminary. The coronary orifices of the graft were adapted to the native ostia and sutured side-to-side. The aorta was closed with a double suture line: mattress and single running stitches. This technique prevents immediate valve regurgitation caused by leaflets or commissure distortion.

From among 126 patients with ascending aortic aneurysm 74 received homografts. The technique of implantation is similar to our 'short cylinder graft' insertion but the allograft is longer and comprises total ascending aorta including valve and distal part adjacent to the brachiocephalic branch. We call it the 'long cylinder graft' (Figs. 1 and 2). The coronary ostia of the graft and of the recipient

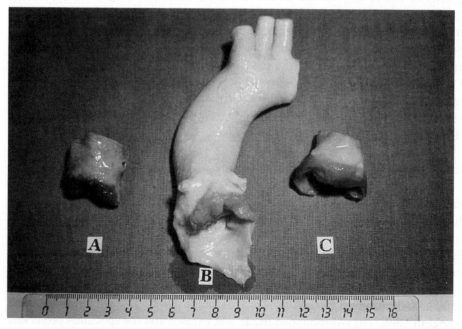

Fig. 1. A, short cylinder graft; B, long cylinder graft; C, pulmonary cylinder.

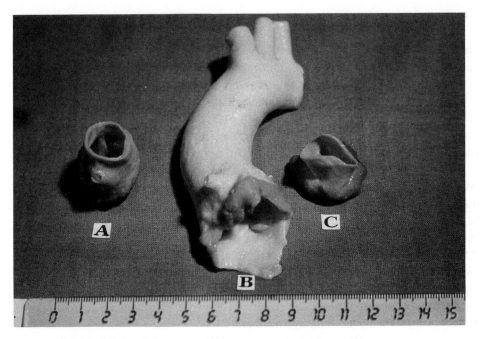

Fig. 2. A, short cylinder graft; B, long cylinder graft; C, pulmonary cylinder.

are carefully adapted and anastomosed side-to-side, and/or, mainly the left coronary, end-to-side, after circle excision and dissection of the ostium from aneurysmatic aortic wall. An additional 3 or 4 single reinforcing sutures are placed around the coronary anastomoses to release the tension of coronary junction and to prevent rupture and bleeding. The distal aortic anastomosis is a routine end-to-end or intraluminar telescope anastomosis. To reinforce the suture line against bleeding or tear, the sutures are passed through the externally located fabric felt tape, placed also internally in case of dissection.

In annulo-aortic ectasia the aortic annulus should be constricted by a single or double fabric ring, inserted around the patient's and the graft's annuli with single straight or mattress sutures. The fabric annuli may be circular in shape or as a tape with 3 indicated distances of the graft commissure and finally, after the sutures are placed, they are formed in a closed circle.

The grafts are wrapped with the remaining aneurysmal wall. To avoid blood cumulating under pressure in the resulting dead space a small hole usually was left for venting. When residual bleed was evident, an anastomosis between the dead space and the right appendage was made routinely. For this purpose the right appendage was saved during cannulation.

The homograft was not touched with fingers, sucker, or instruments especially at its intimal level. The patients were almost routinely cannulated for cardiopulmonary bypass through the external iliac artery to avoid cannula insertion into the false lumen at the ascending aorta level.

Results

From among 412 patients with aortic valve allografts (short cylinder graft) the hospital mortality rate was 4.1%. During mean follow-up of 6 yr (1 mth to over 10 yr) the cumulative late mortality was 2.5%.

In 25% of patients there were in echocardiography some thickening of the aortic leaflets; calcification occurred in 9% of patients (with asymptomatic diastolic BP above 60 mmHg) in 10%. Significant dysfunction of valve homograft was found and reoperated in 6% (25 patients).

From among 126 patients with ascending aortic aneurysm replacement 74 were performed with homograft valve and ascending aorta (long cylinder graft). The hospital mortality rate was 2.7%; late mortality was 6.8% at the mean follow-up time of 6 yr. In patients operated urgently because of acute aortic dissection the operative mortality reached 12.9%. Five patients were successfully reoperated on: three for early valve bacterial endocarditis and two for chronically regurgitation due to massive calcifications developed within three years. During the reoperation the inner layer of the implanted ascending aortic homograft was calcified. It was easy to dissect and to remove the calcified tube with incompetent leaflets and to replace it again with the long cylinder graft.

Discussion

The more than 10-yr experience in our Institution favours free-hand antibiotic sterilized allografts as a good substitute for aortic valve and root replacement. The early and late mortality is acceptable and comparable or lower than after mechanical or bioprosthetic valve implantation [5,13,19,23]. The rate and intensification of degenerative changes of the graft and the graft complications are lower than after insertion of bioprostheses [13,19,21]. Recently introduced cryopreservation of homografts needs more time for clinical evaluation. We recommend to use from the same donor a pulmonary homograft valve as well for aortic valve replacement.There is no evident difference between pulmonary and aortic short cylinder graft insertion. The use of pulmonary graft for side-to-side coronary anastomosis is even easier. The most important technical factors influencing the results and further fate of the grafts and patient are: perfect size and geometry of the implant (this enables the short cylinder graft technique), adequate coronary ostia anastomoses and prevention of annular dilatation in anulo-aortic-ectasia. Our technique of constricting and reinforcing of the annulus using non expandable fabric rings or tapes [12] is essential for the following reasons: it diminishes the risk of bleeding by sutures cutting the tissue, it constricts the grossly widened aortic annulus and it protects the homograft against possible later annulo-aortic ectasia as observation of the patients for more than 6 yr postoperatively confirms.

In our experience, the temporary shunt anastomosis between the dead space around the homograft wrapped with remnant of the aneurysmatic wall and the right atrial appendage may prevent major blood loss and release the tension on the coronary anastomoses [6]. No late shunts were observed.

The importance of the careful completion of the left coronary artery insertion into the graft is emphasized [13,20,22]. Any leakage from this site once the patient is weaned off cardiopulmonary bypass is almost beyond control.

In our opinion, the homografts are of great value in cases with active bacterial endomyocarditis, especially with severe tissue damage with deep abscesses, when the implantation of a prosthetic valve is difficult and connected with high risk of perivalvular leak. If these complications occur, the symptoms develop rapidly. In contrast, the possible dysfunction of the homograft develops gradually and there is much more time for medication and preparation for surgery.

References

1. Al-Yanabi N, Ross DN (1973) Cardiovasc Res 7: 817.
2. Barratt-Boyes BG (1965) Br J Surg 52: 847.
3. Beddermann C, Norman JC, Cooley DA (1980) Cardiovasc Surgeon 29: 89-95.
4. Bentall HH, DeBono A (1968) Thorac 23: 338.
5. Bodnar E, Wain WH, Martelli V, Ross DN (1979) Thorac Cardiovasc Surg 27: 31.
6. Cabrol C, Pavie A, Gandjbakhch I, Villemot JP, Guiraudon G, Langhlin L, Etievent P, Cham B (1981) J Thorac Cardiovasc Surg 81: 309-315.
7. Cooley DA, DeBakey ME (1956) J Am Med Assoc 162: 1159.
8. DeBakey ME, McCollum CH, Crawford ES, Morris GC Jr, Howell J, Noon GP, Lawrie G (1982) Surgery 92: 1118-1134.
9. Detrano R, Moodie DS, Gill CC, Markovich D, Simpfendorfer C (1985) Chest 88: 249.
10. Dziatkowiak AJ, Moll JW, Tracz WD, et al. (1978) Proc 27 Int Congr Eur Soc Cardiovasc Surgeons Lyon, 373.
11. Dziatkowiak AJ, Pfitzner R, Andres J, Podolec P, Marek Z, Zarska M (1988) In: AC Yankah et al., eds. Cardiac Valve Allografts 1962-1987. Darmstadt: Steinkopff Verlag, 141-147.
12. Dziatkowiak AJ, Pfitzner R, Sadowski J, Tracz WD, Koziorowska B, Marek Z (1986) In: E Zacny, E Bodnar and M Yacoub, eds. Biologic and Bioprosthetic Valves, Vol 3. Yorke Medical Books, 14-21.
13. Dziatkowiak AJ, Tracz WD, Sadowski J, Pfitzner R, Koziorowska B, Podolec P (1983) J Cardiovasc Surg 24: 374.
14. Fontan F, Choussat A, Deville C, et al. (1984) J Thorac Cardiovasc Surg 87: 649.
15. Grey DP, Ott DA, Cooley DA (1983) J Thorac Cardiovasc Surg 86: 864-877.
16. Lemole GM, Strong MD, Spagna PM, Karmilowicz NP (1982) J Thorac Cardiovasc Surg 83: 249-255.
17. Massimo CG, Presenti LF, Favi PP, Duranti A, Poma AG, Marranci P, Modiano C (1987) Texas Heart Inst J 14: 418-421.
18. Miller DG, Stinson EB, Oyer, et al. (1980) J Thorac Cardiovasc Surg 79: 388.
19. Penta A, Qureshi J, Radley-Smith R, et al. (1984) Circulation 70 (Suppl. 1).
20. Sadowski J, Dziatkowiak A, Pfitzner R, Tracz W, Kapelak B, Traczyński K (1986) In: G Schlag and H Redl, eds. Sealant in Operative Medicine. Thoracic Surgery, Cardiovascular Surgery, Vol 5. Berlin: Springer Verlag, 201-204.
21. Sommerville J, Ross DN (1982) Br Heart J 47: 473.
22. Thomps, Yacoub M, Ahmed M, Somerville W, Towers M (1980) J Thorac Cardiovasc Surg 79: 896.

158

23. Wheat MW Jr (1980) Am Heart J 99: 373–387.
24. Yacoub M, Kittle CE (1970) Circulation 41 (Suppl. II): 29.

© 1992 Elsevier Science Publishers B.V. All rights reserved
Cardio-thoracic surgery. K. Minami et al. editors.

Hospital-based homograft valve bank

Rudolf Mair, Gerhard Wimmer-Greinecker, Christoph Groß, Wolfgang
Harringer, Peter Hartl and Peter Brücke
I. Surgical Department, AKH Linz, Krankenhausstr. 9, 4020 Linz/D, Austria

Since 1988 we have run a homograft transplant program in our department.
Allograft valves can be obtained from international valve banks, but complex
transport organisation, low flexibility in graft selection and dependence on an
organisation far away from our department are severe disadvantages. Therefore
we believe that the frequent use of allograft valves suggests a hospital-based
valve bank [1].

A prerequisite for a successful homograft bank is the recruitment of enough
homograft donors. The following criteria are posited: age between 3 and 55 yr;
no malignant disease; no signs of sepsis, lues, hepatitis, AIDS or slow virus
disease; no penetrating thoracic trauma; no previous cardiac procedures.

The number of donors in our hospital would be too small to cover our own
supply. Therefore we cooperate with various clinics and transplant institutions.
They are listed in Table 1 together with the corresponding number of donor
hearts.

Our donors are transplant recipients (35%), brain-dead organ donors (32%) and
cadaver donors (33%). Cadaver donors are only accepted within 24 h after
cardiac arrest as long as the cadaver is stored in a refrigerator between 0 and 4°C.
The hearts are explanted under sterile conditions by surgeons. Some blood
samples are taken at that time for serologic and virologic investigations (see
Table 2). The heart is kept in lactated Ringer's solution covered with ice and
brought into the operating room, where the valves are prepared.

The ascending aorta and the aortic arch as well as the pulmonary artery are
preserved as long as possible; the coronaries are ligated; the anterior mitral leaflet
stays in continuity with the aortic homograft; the subanular part of the ventricular
myocardium is cut circularly without scalloping along the base of the cusps; the
adventitia of the great arteries is preserved; the diameter of the valve is measured
by a conic sizer, and the valve competence is tested.

The posterior mitral leaflet is used for microbiological investigations.

After preparation the valves are sterilised in an antibiotic solution ([2] see
Table 3), where they are kept at body temperature for 6 h and at 0 to 4°C for a
further 18 h. After sterilisation two specimens are taken for a second microbiological investigation. The valve is then brought into tissue culture medium RPMI
1640 containing human albumin up to a concentration of 10% (90 ml); 10 ml of
dimethyl sulphoxide are added. Allografts and solution are packed in polyole-
phine bags (Gambro DF 1200), using an impulse-heat-sealer. After 2 h the valves

Table 1. Donor centers

MH Hannover	69
II. Chir.Univ.Klinik, Wien	37
I. Chir.Univ.Klinik, Wien	34
Wagner-Jauregg-KH, Linz	15
Wels	11
UKH Linz	9
LKH Salzburg	7
Kirchdorf/Krems	6
KH Elisabethinen, Linz	2
Gmünd	2
Vöcklabruck	2
I. Chir.Univ.Klinik, Innsbruck	1
Ried	1
Bad Ischl	1
LKH Klagenfurt	1
AKH Linz	45
Total	243

undergo a controlled freezing procedure down to −40°C valve temperature (dT/dt = 1°C/min). For this procedure we use a computerized freezer (Ice cube 1610, Sylab). Finally the valves are stored in liquid nitrogen.

So far preparation, sterilization and freezing have been done by the staff surgeons of our department. As the number of banked valves will increase we will have to employ a medical technician especially for sterilizing, freezing and administrative issues.

Table 2. Serology and virology

Blood group, rhesus factor
Syphilis
Hepatitis B, hepatitis C
HIV

Table 3. Sterilization

Antibiotic solution:	polimyxine B 10 mg/100 ml
	vancomycin 10 mg/100 ml
	cefoxitin 24 mg/100 ml
	lincomycin 12 mg/100 ml
	amphotericin B 2.5 mg/100 ml

+ RPMI 1640 and 10% human albumin (50 ml) throughout 24 h

If a valve is requested, it is thawed rapidly at 37°C until sludge occurs, then DMSO is diluted in 4 steps. If another clinic calls for an allograft, they are sent in dry ice by train or plane to many destinations in Europe.

Up to now we have implanted 101 aortic and 54 pulmonary allografts in aortic position and performed 17 autografts. We believe that we could never have reached this amount of implanted homograft valves without our own valve bank.

References

1. Lange PL, Hopkins RA (1989) Allograft valve banking – techniques and technology. In: RA Hopkins, ed. Cardiac Reconstruction with Allograft Valves, Ch 4. Berlin: Springer Verlag.
2. Heacox AE, Mcnally RT, Rockbank KGM (1987) Factors affecting the viability of cryo-preserved allograft heart valves. In: AC Yankah, R Hetzer, BC Mill, J Somerwille, MH Yacoub and DN Ross, eds. Cardiac Valve Allografts 1962–1987. Current Concept on the Use of Aortic and Pulmonary Allografts for Heart Valve Substitute. Steinkopf Verlag, Springer Verlag.

© 1992 Elsevier Science Publishers B.V. All rights reserved
Cardio-thoracic surgery. K. Minami et al. editors.

163

Surgical treatment of Wolff-Parkinson-White syndrome

T. Iwa, T. Misaki, Y. Matsunaga and M. Tsubota

Department of Surgery, Kanazawa University School of Medicine, Takaramachi 13-1, Kanazawa 920, Japan

Introduction

Since 1969, when we performed the first original atrial endocardial approach for Wolff-Parkinson-White (WPW) syndrome [1], we have operated on more than 600 various tachyarrhythmias at Sapporo Medical College Hospital, Kanazawa University Hospital, and several other hospitals in Japan. This communication is based on this accumulated experience and the complete data available for the 433 consecutive cases of WPW syndrome operated on at Kanazawa University Hospital between May 1, 1973, and March 31, 1991.

Development of surgical method for WPW syndrome

Sealy et al. [2] successfully treated a case of WPW syndrome in 1968 using an epicardial right ventricular incision to exclude the pre-excitation site. In 1969, Iwa et al. [1] originated an incision of the right atrium from only the endocardial side along the tricuspid annulus for the WPW syndrome. Later in 1974, Sealy [3] changed his approach from an epicardial and ventricular one to an endocardial and atrial one after performing his epicardial approach in 10 cases. Our method involved less dissection of the area of the atrioventricular (A-V) groove than that of Sealy. We did not dissect the atrial side at all (Fig. 1). We believe that the accessory pathway (AP) is located on the outer side of the atrial muscle, close to the annular ring and not in the fat tissue of the A-V groove. Cox et al. [4] followed Sealy's method generally, but possibly their dissection of the A-V groove was more extensive and systematic. Thus, the endocardial atrial approach has become the standard surgical method for WPW syndrome.

Gallagher et al. [5] introduced the epicardial use of cryoablation for WPW syndrome in 1977. We added cryoablation almost routinely after interruption of the atrium between 1982 and 1987 [6] and it is being used at present only for septal AP. Gallagher's epicardial cryoablation was not subsequently used by his own group, while Guiraudon extended the use of cryoablation epicardially with or without heart-lung bypass [7,8].

At present, after gaining considerable experience and regardless of whether the approach is endocardial or epicardial, surgical treatment can achieve excellent results in almost all cases of WPW syndrome.

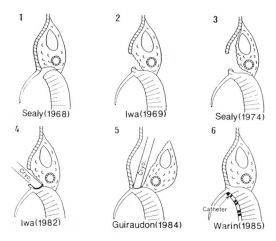

Fig. 1. Surgical methods.

Indications for surgery

The indications for surgery have remained unchanged since the operation was first developed [9]. They are: (1) ventricular fibrillation or atrial fibrillation with rapid ventricular response, (2) short effective refractory period less than 250 ms, (3) refractory to medication, (4) severe complaints (e.g. faintness, nausea, dizziness), (5) combined heart disease to be operated on, (6) poor hemodynamic state during tachycardia (e.g. hypotension, low cardiac output, shock), and (7) need for long-term medication. However, as the safety and reliability of surgical intervention have improved, surgery has been extended to patients showing somewhat less serious symptoms, and the number of such patients has been increasing.

Table 1. Concurrent heart disease

Congenital	No. of patients	Acquired	No. of patients
Ebstein's anomaly	40	Angina pectoris	10
Anterior tricuspid annular dysplasia (10)	10	Cardiomyopathy	7
		Mitral stenosis	6
Atrial septal defect	2	Mitral regurgitation	3
Tricuspid atresia	2	Aortic stenosis	1
VSD + PDA	1	Combined valvular disease	3
Left superior vena cava	1	Annuloaortic ectasia	1
Corrected transportion + PS	1	Idiopathic tricuspid	
Endocardial cushion defect	1	regurgitation	1
Total	58		32

Cases

A total of 433 patients, 311 male and 122 female, received operation for WPW syndrome at the Kanazawa University Hospital from all over Japan and 3 cases from abroad. They ranged in age from 5 mth to 74 yr, with a mean age of 37.2 + 15.9 yr, including 21 cases of small children less than 10 yr old.

Concurrent heart diseases were noted in 89 patients (20.6%), these consisted of 57 congenital, 31 acquired, and one congenital (Ebstein's anomaly) combined with acquired disease (annuloaortic ectasia) (Table 1). Ebstein's anomaly was the most common combined heart disease and it was found in 40 patients. Concurrent heart diseases were surgically treated simultaneously with the WPW syndrome in 64 patients, excluding patients in whom operation was not indicated.

Preoperative examination

Routine preoperative studies included 12-lead electrocardiography, vectorcardiography, echocardiography, nuclear cardiography, body surface mapping, and a clinical cardiac electrophysiological study. All these procedures have been detailed previously [10]. To locate the ACP, all these techniques are useful with different grades of certainty [11]. In particular, the 12-lead electrocardiogram by Iwa's criteria (Table 2) was the simplest but most accurate examination [9,11,12].

During the surgery, complete epicardial mapping of both ventricles has not been used since the introduction of a simple catheter electrode method in 1982 [10,13]. Electrical potentials at 6 points and a reference lead are measured simultaneously using a multibipolar electrode catheter applied on a ventricle at the A-V groove. The earliest preexcitation site can be identified at a glance. The earliest excitation site of the atrium during tachycardia or rapid ventricular pacing was also studied to detect the insertion site of AP into the atrium. Usually, it was found at the contralateral site of the earliest preexcitation site of the ventricle.

Table 2. Iwa's criteria [9,11] for localizing the AP in 8 regions by polarity of the delta wave

RFW	V1 (±)
RAW	III, aVF (+)
RLW	III, aVF (variate in between)
RPW	III, aVF (−)
RS	V1 (−)
RAS	III, aVF (+)
RPS	III, aVF (−)
Left	V1 (+)
LAW	III, aVF (+)
LLW	I (+) or (−), aVL (−)
LPW	III, aVF (−)
LPS	III, aVF (−)

Surgical method

The surgical method used has been consistently atrial endocardial incision, to which cryoablation was added in 1982, although it has been applied only for septal AP after 1988 or case No. 300. In most of the cases, the operation was performed without blood prime for heart-lung bypass to avoid serum hepatitis.

Left cardiac type

After exposing the mitral orifice, the stay suture placed earlier at the pre-excitation site of the left ventricle is palpated with a finger on the endocardium of the left atrium and the position is marked with another stay suture on the atrial endocardium. An incision starting from this point and extending 2–3 cm on both sides of the mark is made with a scalpel on the wall of the left atrial endocardium along the mitral ring 2 mm apart and is deepened until the fatty tissue of the A-V groove appears. Although the atrial wall is very thin, 1–2 mm, in the normal heart, the wall near the AP is frequently thickened in the WPW syndrome due to abnormal stimulation and excitation. Such thickening is especially remarkable in older patients who have experienced frequent attacks of tachycardia. Since the AP is closely adjacent to the cardiac muscle, adjunctive sites between the incised atrial rim, mitral annulus and earliest pre-exciting ventricle are dissected intentionally with an angled knife (Beaver 5610). The 1.0–1.5 cm wide left ventricular muscle from the anulus is disclosed by the dissection. The incised atrial rim of the distal atrial side is not dissected from the fatty tissue at all (Fig. 1). The incised atrial rim is carefully reapproximated with a continuous 4-0 Prolene suture.

Right cardiac type

In the right cardiac type, the interruption is made while the heart is beating during heart-lung bypass after closing the foramen ovale if it is patent. Therefore, interruption of the AP can be confirmed by the disappearance of the delta wave on the electrocardiogram monitor. The ECG pattern is normalized when the AP is divided. Dissection of the A-V adjunctive area is identical to that of the left cardiac type.

In the case of a right septal AP, the normal conduction system located close to the AP is identified based on anatomical knowledge and a His bundle electrogram using the catheter electrode. The dissection is more difficult than that for a free wall AP because there is often no fatty tissue between the atrium and ventricle in the right septal area, and the atrium is attached to the ventricle forming a plane rather a line like in the free wall. The incision is similarly made, 2 mm apart and along the tricuspid ring. Additional cryoablation is often employed at the site of disappearance of the delta wave to ensure complete ablation, while the His bundle electrogram is being monitored by an electrode in order to avoid the creation of A-V block (Fig. 2).

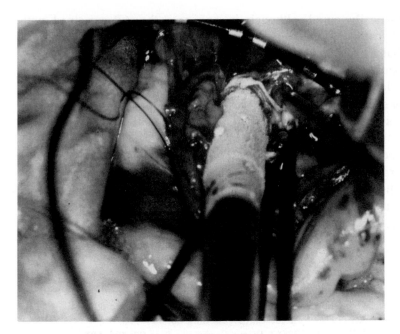

Fig. 2. See the text.

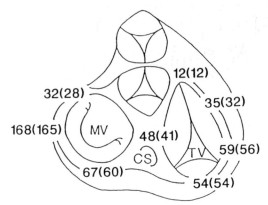

Total ACPs : 475 (448)

Fig. 3. Localization of AP. Free-standing numbers indicate APs confirmed by epicardial mapping in 433 patients. Parentheses contain the number of successfully interrupted APs. One patient had 3 APs in different sites.

Surgical results

APs were successfully ablated in 407 of the 433 patients (94.0%) received surgical treatment (Fig. 3). Interruption was incomplete in 26 patients, but paroxysmal tachycardia did not appear or appeared only a few times in 25 of 26 patients during the long follow-up period and so these patients were considered

168

to be symptomatically cured, although in one case the AP remained with paroxysmal tachycardia. There were 41 cases with multiple APs, excluding 4 cases with Mahaim's fibers. One of the multiple APs remained in the 12 cases without tachycardia attack postoperatively. They were included in the above 25 failure cases. Eleven patients died from 1 to 33 days (mean 7 days) postoperatively after successful interruption of APs. All these patients had concurrent cardiac disease, simultaneously operated on, and died of causes other than WPW syndrome.

In the most recent 169 consecutive cases, we have achieved an almost 100% success rate characterized by no recurrence, no reoperation, no A-V block and no deaths. One of the multiple APs has remained in the 4 cases without tachycardia attack. Exceptionally, late death due to renal failure occurred in one patient 3 mth after the surgery.

References

1. Iwa T, Kazui T, Sugii S, et al. (1970) Jpn J Thor Surg 23: 513-518.
2. Sealy WC, Hattler BG Jr, Blumenschein SD, et al. (1969) Ann Thor Surg 8: 1-11.
3. Sealy WC, Wallace AG (1974) J Thorac Cardiovasc Surg 68: 757-770.
4. Cox JL, Gallagher JJ, Cain ME (1985) J Thorac Cardiovasc Surg 90: 490-501.
5. Gallagher JJ, Sealy WC, Anderson RW, et al. (1977) Circulation 55: 471-479.
6. Iwa T, Misaki T, Iida S (1983) J Cardiovasc Surg 24: 447 (Abstr).
7. Guiraudon GM, Klein GJ, Sharma AD (1986) Ann Thorac Surg 42: 651-657.
8. Guiraudon GM, Klein GJ, Yee R, et al. (1990) Ann Thorac Surg 50: 968-971.
9. Iwa T, Kawasuji M, Misaki T, et al. (1980) J Thorac Cardiovasc Surg 80: 271-279.
10. Iwa T, Mukai K, Misaki T, et al. (1988) In: T Iwa and G Fontaine, eds. Cardiac Arrhythmias. Recent Progress in Investigation and Management. Amsterdam: Elsevier, 241-250.
11. Yuan S, Iwa T, Misaki T, et al. (in press) Jpn Circul J (in press).
12. Yuan S, Iwa T, Tsubota, et al. (in press).
13. Mitsui T, Iwa T, Kitamura A (1983) Jpn J Thoracic Surg 36: 716-718.

Surgical treatment of life-threatening ventricular arrythmias after myocardial infarction

V. Dor[1], M. Sabatier[1], M. Di Donato[2], F. Bourlon[1], P. Rossi[1], T. Lanzillo[1] and F. Montiglio[1]

[1]Cardiothoracic Center, 11 bis Avenue d'Ostende, 98000 Principauté de Monaco and
[2]Department of Cardiology, University of Florence, Italy

Introduction

Surgery has become an important form of treatment for life-threatening ventricular arrythmias in patients (pts) with coronary artery disease (CAD) and severe left ventricular (LV) wall motion abnormalities, mainly LV aneurysm. Standard aneurysmectomy, alone or in combination with coronary bypass surgery, has not been consistently effective in abolishing malignant ventricular arrythmias.

Since 1985 we have adopted an original technique of left ventricular reconstruction consisting in endoventricular circular patch plasty after extended endocardectomy [1-3] for the treatment of postinfarction dyskinetic or akinetic LV aneurysm. We designed this study in order to evaluate the efficacy of such surgical technique in abolishing spontaneous or inducible, sustained LV tachycardia (VT) in pts with previous myocardial infarction and severe LV wall motion abnormalities. For this purpose each patient had pre- and postoperative programmed right ventricular stimulation. The present paper focuses on the results obtained in 41 pts out of 110 who had spontaneous or inducible VT.

Methods

Study patients
Between 1989 and June 1991, 110 consecutive pts with postinfarction LV akinetic or dyskinetic aneurysm and CAD have undergone surgical treatment at the Monte Carlo Cardiothoracic Center. There were 101 males and 9 females with a mean age of 57 ± 7 yr.

Preoperative evaluation: each pt underwent complete angiographic and hemodynamic study including coronary arteriography and LV angiography. Pts with acute myocardial infarction were excluded. Pts had at least one coronary stenosis that occluded more than 75% of the artery. Programmed right ventricular electrical stimulation (PVS) was performed with the following protocol: (1) apex ventricular pacing from 100 to 200 bpm; (2) single or double extra-stimulus introduced after 8 ventricular beats at a cycle length of 600 and 500 ms. A third extra-stimulus was given if VT was clinically detected. The goal of electrophysiologic test was limited to the induction of monomorphic VT lasting

170

more than 15 s. Induced VT was terminated by overdrive pacing, paired extra-
beats or external cardioversion. No serious complication occurred during the
protocol.

Postoperative evaluation: patients underwent complete hemodynamic and
angiographic study early after surgery (8–15 days).

Table 1 shows pre- and postoperative electrophysiologic studies. Early PVS
was performed off antiarrythmic drugs. Ninety-six pts completed the protocol of
PVS before and early after surgery; 7 pts with spontaneous VT and severely
impaired LV function had PVS performed only after surgery (Table 1).

Pts were discharged from antiarrythmic drugs except pts with spontaneous or
inducible postsurgery VT, who were given Amiodarone.

Thirty-two pts had complete hemodynamic study including PVS at 1 yr after
surgery; clinical follow-up is available for 31 pts from 3 to 14 mth.

Surgical technique

Left ventricular reconstruction (LVR) by endoventricular patch plasty, with septal
exclusion, consists in attaching inside the left ventricle (LV) a circular piece of
synthetic or autologous tissue, which allows one to exclude all akinetic non-
resectable areas in addition to the aneurysmal area that has been resected or
folded in the classical way.

The akinetic or aneurysmal area is easily detected when it collapses after
aspiration of the bulb. It is vertically incised forward and beyond the apex. The
fibrous, cicatricial endocardium is dissected from the ventricular wall, that is from
the fibrous remaining epicardium and myocardium; the mural thrombi are
mobilized and extracted at the same time. This dissection is extended far into the
left ventricular wall, to the healthy area of the septum inside, to the papillary
muscle root at the back and above and to the healthy myocardium outside. The
endocardial tissue is resected and if there is any ventricular tachycardia, cryotherapy is used on the edges of this resection. A prolene 2/0 wire is basted in a

Table 1. Pre- and postoperative electrophysiologic studies

	Pre	Post (early)	Post (late)
Pts studied	96	102	32
Pts not studied	14	8	78
EF < 20%	5	0	
Spontaneous VT or VF	7	2	
Other reasons	2	3	
Perioperative death		2	
Cardiac transplantation		1	
Total pts	110	110	

Early = 9–12 days post-surgery; late = 1 yr post-surgery.

circle at this resection's limit (Jatene-Fontan method) and a patch of the size of this endoventricular opening is prepared: Dacron lined with pericardium or pieces of fibrous septal endocardium, mobilized on a septal hinge if this endocardium is resistant with no calcification or mural thrombus. This piece is attached to the contractile endo-ventricular edge by a continuous suture resting on a pericardial splint. The excluded epicardial and myocardial edges can be resected but more often folded over the patch in order to reinforce it as well as the hemostasis. The detailed surgical technique has been reported in our previous works [1–3].

Results

The patient population is reported in Table 2. Pre- and postoperative electrophysiologic data are reported in Table 3.

Preoperative results

Mean EF was $39 \pm 14\%$. There was a total of 54 episodes of spontaneous ($n = 20$) and/or inducible VT ($n = 34$). All pts with spontaneous arrythmias who underwent PVS had inducible VT ($n = 13$); VT was induced in 21 pts without preoperative spontaneous arrythmias (23%).

Table 2. Patient population ($n = 110$), 101 males; 9 females; mean age 57 ± 7 yr

	n
CAD	110
ANASA	96
AKINASA	10
POSTAN	4

Abbreviations: CAD = coronary artery disease; ANASA = aneurysm anteroseptoapical; AKINASA = akinesy anteroseptoapical; POSTAN = posterior aneurysm.

Table 3. Pre- and postoperative ventricular arrythmias in 41 pts

	Pre (n)	Post (early) (n)	Post (late) (n)
	110	108	32
Spont VF	3	0	0
Spont VT	17	2	0
Induced VT	34	6	1

Abbreviations: VF = ventricular fibrillation; VT = ventricular tachycardia.

Table 4. Operative procedure

	Pts (*n*)
LV reconstruction with septal exclusion	110
Associated procedures:	
CABG	108
Endocardectomy	51
Endocardectomy + cryotherapy	15 (66)
Perioperative mortality	2

Abbreviation: CABG = coronary artery bypass grafting.

Table 5. Pre- and postoperative ejection fraction (EF)

	EF %
Preoperative	39 ± 14
Postoperative (early)	49 ± 13*
Postoperative (late)	49 ± 14*

*$p < 0.01$
Early = 9–12 days post-surgery; late = 1 yr post-surgery.

Postoperative results

Operative procedure is reported in Table 4. Perioperative mortality was 1.8%. EF significantly increased after surgery (Table 5) and end diastolic volume index significantly decreased (from $117 ± 47$ to $81 ± 24$ ml/m^2). VT was induced in 6 pts, 2 of whom had preop inducible VT; thus 32 out of 34 pts with preop inducible VT (94%) had no inducible VT after surgery (Fisher's exact test, $p < 0.001$). One of the 20 pts with preop spontaneous VT had postop spontaneous arrythmias.

No predictive variable has been found by discriminant analysis; however, pts with preoperative inducible VT had significantly lower EF ($35 ± 12$% vs. $41 ± 15$%, $p < 0.05$).

At 1 yr clinical control, there has been no hospitalization for life-threatening arrythmias since surgery.

Discussion

LV aneurysmectomy and bypass grafting are widely used to treat malignant ventricular arrythmias but the results have not been uniform [4–7]. Several factors influence the results, including (1) type of arrythmias; (2) the temporal relationship of the arrythmias to the ischemic events; and (3) varying surgical technique. There is evidence that standard aneurysmectomy, alone or in combination with bypass grafting, fails to abolish the arrythmias because it rarely removes the segment of the border and almost never the septal segment of the aneurism, a site which is often the origin of VT [8–10].

Better results have been obtained with intraoperative guided endocardial resection [11–14]; however, this technique is time-consuming and has major limitations. Other publications have demonstrated that non-guided endocardial resection gives good results for the treatment of sustained, spontaneous VT [15].

Our technique allows exclusion of the akinetic septum and, by means of circular reorganization of the remaining muscle, it allows one to achieve a 'more physiological cavity', with improvement of EF (see Table 5). Moreover, endo-cardectomy performed in the majority of pts with inducible or spontaneous VT, cryotherapy at the border of the lesion, together with a complete myocardial revascularization, are all factors that can play a role in the success in abolishing the arrythmias in our series of patients. Two problems concerning ventricular arrythmias and coronary artery disease have to be discussed, in our opinion:

(1) The prognostic significance of inducible VT, in the absence of clinically, spontaneous malignant arrhythmias, has been questioned since natural history studies have not been completed; however, a recent paper by Nogami et al. [16] clearly shows that programmed ventricular stimulation after 1 mth from myocardial infarction has significant predictive value for sudden cardiac death and for sustained ventricular tachyarrythmias.

(2) Data from the literature have shown that the extended endocardial resection procedure associated with aneurysmectomy has considerable risks of death or of deterioration of LV function [17–19].

Our results demonstrate that the overall mortality rate is very low in this series of pts with the described technical procedure; moreover, a significant increase in pump function has been obtained after surgery as well as a significant decrease of spontaneous and inducible VT occurrence.

It is well known that EF is an independent predictor of survival in coronary artery disease; moreover, an EF less than 40% coupled with the presence of the LV aneurysm is a predictor of malignant ventricular arrythmias [20]. Therefore, we believe that the surgical technique here described, by resecting the aneurysm and by improving LV pump function, can improve the prognosis of these patients, in terms of both survival and arrhythmia-free events. In this respect, our results at 1 yr, even if not completed, seem encouraging. A long-term follow-up on a larger series of patients is needed to confirm the results.

We conclude that the 'aggressive' way of approaching the treatment of postinfarction LV aneurysm with malignant ventricular arrythmias can be safely performed and provides good early results in terms of improved LV function and reduced malignant arrythmias.

174

References

1. Dor V, Bourlon F, Sabatier M, Grinneiser D, Montiglio F, Coste P, Saab M, Rossi P (1990) Arch Mal Coeur 83: 1657-1694.
2. Dor V (1990) Current opinion in cardiology. Current science ISSN 0268-4705.
3. Dor V, Jourdan J, Coste P, Viglione J, Saab M, Grinneiser D, Bourlon F, Sabatier M, Montiglio F (1989) Cardiac Reconstruction. Berlin: Springer Verlag.
4. Sami M, Chaitma BR, Bourassa MG, Charpin D, Chabot M (1978) Am Heart J 96: 303-307.
5. Thind GS, Blakemore WS, Zinsser HP (1971) Am J Cardiol 27: 690-694.
6. Harken AH, Horowitz LN, Josephson ME (1980) J Thorac Cardiovasc Surg 80: 527.
7. Ricks WB, Winkle RA, Shumway NG, Harrison DC (1977) Circulation 56: 38-42.
8. Sealy WC, Oldham HN (1978) In: DT Kelley, ed. Advances in the Management of Arrythmias. Australia, Télectronics, 218-224.
9. Miller JM, Kienzle MG, Harken AH, Josephson ME (1984) Circulation 706: 624-631.
10. Wiener I, Mindich B, Pitchon R (1982) Circulation 65: 856-861.
11. Horowitz LN, Harken AH, Kastor JA, Josephson ME (1980) N Engl J Med 302: 589-593.
12. Josephson ME, Harken AH, Horowitz LN (1979) Circulation 60: 1430-1439.
13. Harken AH, Josephson ME, Horowitz LN (1979) Ann Surg 190: 456-460.
14. Josephson ME, Harken AH, Horowitz LN (1982) Am Heart J 104: 51-57.
15. Zee-Cheng CS, Kouchoukos NT, Connors JP, Ruffy R (1989) JACC 13: 153-162.
16. Nogami A, Aounuma K, Takahashi A, Nitta J, Chun YH, Iesaka Y, Hiroe M, Marumo F (1991) Am J Cardiol 68: 13-20.
17. Kowey PR, Friehling TD, Marinchak RA (1989) Am J Cardiol 64: 832 (Letter).
18. Garan H, Nguyen K, McGovern B, Buckley M, Ruskin JN (1986) JACC 8: 201-209.
19. Miller JM, Gottlieb CD, Hargrove WC, Josephson ME (1981) Circulation 78 (Suppl. II): 11-44.
20. Furukawa T, Rozanski JJ, Moroe K, Gosselin AJ, Lister JW (1989) Am Heart J 117: 1050-1059.

175

Implantable cardioverter defibrillators in the treatment of malignant ventricular arrhythmia

G.H. Almassi, G.N. Olinger, J. Veseth-Rogers, J.N. Wetherbee and
P.D. Chapman
*Department of Cardiothoracic Surgery, Medical College of Wisconsin, 8700 West Wisconsin
Avenue, Milwaukee, WI 53226, U.S.A.*

Introduction

It is estimated that 20% to 30% of patients suffering from sudden cardiac death are successfully resuscitated [1–3]. In the United States, about 400,000 people suffer from sudden cardiac death annually, of whom between 80,000 to 120,000 will survive the sudden cardiac death episode. With medical treatment alone, the annual recurrence rate ranges between 10% and 30% [4–7]. The success of implantable cardioverter defibrillators (ICD) in prolonging the survival of such patients has been proven by our own data and those of other investigators [8–11]. The worldwide acceptance of ICDs as effective therapy for malignant ventricular arrhythmias is evidenced by the remarkable number of defibrillators that have been implanted worldwide over the last three and one-half years (Table 1). Our experience with the implantation of defibrillators began in June 1983, and is reported here through March 1, 1991.

Patient material

Between June 1983 and March 1991, 218 patients (190 male, 28 female) underwent implantation of ICDs at the Medical College of Wisconsin. Twenty-nine other patients had defibrillator patch and sensing lead placement, usually in conjunction with other cardiac surgical procedures and as part of our then staged implantation of ICD protocol [11] and are not included in this report.

Patient demographics are shown in Table 2. The mean age was 61 yr (range 14 to 90). Depressed left ventricular function with ejection fraction < 0.30 was

Table 1. Representative world wide experience with ICD

	1988	1989	1990	1991 (up to June 30)
CPI AICD Implants	7282	11723	18937	23405 (21781 USA)
Ventritex Cadence				442
Total				23847 (22206 USA)

Data provided by: CPI, Inc., St. Paul, MN and Ventritex, Inc., La Jolla, CA, U.S.A.

present in 54% of the patients and in 21% the ejection fraction was < 0.20; 13% were in NYHA Class III and IV. Seventy-six percent of the patients had failed at least three or more antiarrhythmic drugs before the ICD implantation. The indications for ICD implantation are shown in Table 3. Table 4 shows the type of implants received and the number of patients who had permanent pacemaker implants as well. Complete ICD systems were implanted in one stage in 183 patients; 151 patients had ICD alone, 24 patients had concomitant isolated

Table 2. Clinical characteristics

Age:	Mean	61 yr ± 12 yr	
	Range	14 - 90 yr	
Sex:	Male	190 (87%)	
	Female	28 (13%)	
Diagnosis:		CAD	170 (78%)
		Cardiomyopathy	36 (17%)
		Primary electrical disease	6 (3%)
		Others	6 (3%)
Ejection fraction (%) 33.2 ± 15.0			
Failed drugs:		< 3 drugs	52 (24%)
		> 3 drugs	166 (76%)
Arrhythmia:		VT	86 (39%)
		VF	30 (14%)
		Both	102 (47%)

CAD = coronary artery disease, VT = ventricular tachycardia, VF = ventricular fibrillation.

Table 3. Indications for ICD implantation

1. Cardiac arrest and/or hypotensive VT with or without inducible VT at EP study resistant to drug therapy.
2. Cardiomyopathy with depressed ejection fraction and inducible VT at EP study resistant to drug therapy.
3. Bridge to transplantation.

EP = electrophysiology.

Table 4. Type of implanted devices

Type of implant	Number of patients
CPI-AICD	200
Ventritex-Cadence	18 (4 with previous CPI AICDs)
Permanent transvenous pacemaker	24

coronary bypass, 3 patients had surgical ablative procedure, and 5 patients had other cardiac procedures. Staged implantation with leads first was done in 14 patients during isolated coronary bypass, 11 patients during a surgical ablative procedure, and in 10 patients with other cardiac procedures.

Ten patients underwent implantation of ICD as a bridge to transplantation. In this group, one patient developed infection of the device and his system was removed. He subsequently expired from an arrhythmic death at home. All nine other patients subsequently underwent successful cardiac transplantation. Five are presently alive. Three of the four deaths were late after cardiac transplantation (more than 6 mth) and were related to graft rejection. The fourth patient died ultimately from infection present around the defibrillating patch leads at the time of cardiac transplantation at another institution.

Left anterior thoracotomy was the preferred surgical approach for the implantation of ICD (141 patients). When concomitant surgical procedures were being done median sternotomy was used. After discharge from the hospital, the patients were followed in the cardiac arrhythmia clinic according to standard protocol every 1–3 mth.

Other than common postoperative sequelae such as atelectasis and incisional chest pain, the major complications in this series were infections of the implanted devices (5.5%) and fracture of the sensing and/or defibrillating leads. Table 5 shows infectious complications in this series and the causative organisms. Ten patients developed infection of the ICD, necessitating the removal of the whole system. Two patients died following explantation of the system from arrhythmic deaths. Except for one patient who refused a second ICD implant the remainder underwent implantation of a second ICD at a later date. Two additional patients had thickened, fibrotic capsules around the generators that were excised during generator replacement. Cultures from the excised tissue subsequently grew *Staphylococcus epidermidis*. In both cases the systems were left in place and patients were placed on chronic suppressive oral antibiotics. The majority of the infections, whether early or late, were due to *Staphylococcus aureus* or *epidermidis*. Lead complications are listed in Table 6. Fifteen instances of shocking lead replacements occurred in 13 patients. In three patients the shocking lead was fractured and required replacement and in the other 13 instances high defibrillation threshold (DFT) necessitated either replacing the patch lead with a new lead (5 instances), or switching from an intravascular spring lead to an epicardial patch lead system (3 instances) or vice versa (4 instances).

Follow-up ranges from 1 mth to 98 mth with a mean of 35.7 mth and a total of 5562 patient-months. One patient was lost to follow-up 22.6 mth after his initial ICD implantation. Operative mortality was 1.8% (4 patients). Device failure to terminate intractable ventricular tachycardia and fibrillation was the cause of death in one patient. The other two patients died from noncardiac causes. A fourth patient died at home 10 days following ICD implantation from a documented sudden cardiac death and electromechanical dissociation. His device functioned appropriately. Forty-nine other patients died during the follow-up period for an overall mortality of 22.8%. The causes of deaths are listed in Table 7. The actuarial survival of patients is 92% at 1 yr, 85.2% at 2 yr, 66% at 5 yr, and 47.8% at 7 yr. Patients with LV ejection fraction > 0.3 had a better long-term survival than patients with a more depressed LV function (72.8% 5 yr survival vs. 56%, $p = 0.004$ log rank test). Similarly the survival of patients on less than three antiarrhythmic drugs at the time of device implantation was significantly better than those patients on more than three drugs (90.4% vs. 60.6% 5 yr survival, $p = 0.018$ log rank test).

Table 5. ICD infective complications

Patient Age (yr)	Organisms	Interval to infection (months)	ICD Explant	ICD Reimplant	Follow-up
72	Gram-positive cocci	18	yes	yes	Alive and well
31	*Staph. aureus*	1	yes	no	Dead at 2 wk (SCD)
64	*Staph. epidermidis*	1	yes	no	Dead (SCD)
49	*Staph. aureus*	3	yes	yes	Dead at 3 mth of Serratia sepsis
66	*Staph. epidermidis*	2	yes	no	Alive and well
68	*Staph. aureus*	4	yes	yes	Dead at 2 yr from pneu- monia
60	*Staph. aureus*	1	yes	yes	Dead at 5 mth from P.E.
63	Mixed *Staph. epidermidis* *Staph. aureus* *Strep. faecalis*	1	yes	yes	Alive and well
70	*Staph. aureus*	5	yes	yes	Alive and well
48	*Staph. epidermidis*	26	yes	N/A	Dead at 4 mth post-transplant
72	*Staph. epidermidis*	29	no	N/A	Alive and well
63	*Staph. epidermidis*	24	no	N/A	Alive and well

P.E. = pulmonary embolus, SCD = sudden cardiac death.

Table 6. Lead complications

	Sensing Lead	Defibrillating Lead
Fracture	11	3
High DFT	NA	12
Poor R-wave	4	NA
Infection	10	10

DFT = defibrillating threshold.

Table 8 shows the number of shocks or antitachycardia pacing episodes (ATP) that have occurred in these patients. Propriety of the episodes are defined as: Appropriate – the event was documented by telemetry, holter monitoring, or was associated with the loss of consciousness that was witnessed or was confirmed by electrogram; Inappropriate – documented by telemetry or holter monitoring, or was reproducible by arm movement, exercise, or lead fracture was confirmed; Unknown – all other events even if symptoms of lightheadedness or presyncope were present.

In those patients who had the Ventritex V100 (Cadence) antitachycardia defibrillator system, 210 episodes of appropriate conversion of tachycardia were recorded and 426 episodes of antitachycardia pacing were of unknown propriety. Seventeen episodes were judged by intracardiac electrogram inappropriate. In this category, one patient who had multiple episodes of shocks with a CPI AICD underwent conversion of this unit to a Cadence. He subsequently had 69 episodes of antitachycardia pacing arrhythmic conversion appropriately, and 336 episodes of antitachycardia pacing that were of unknown propriety where the device was functioning to convert a presumably arrhythmic episode. There has been no DC shock with this system in this patient. Of the 18 patients in this series who had the Cadence system implanted, four had a CPI ICD initially which was subsequently converted to a Cadence V100 device.

Implantation of a CPI Endotak lead system (the non-thoracotomy system) was

Table 7. Causes of death

	Number of deaths
Arrhythmic (sudden and non sudden)	11
Cardiac nonarrhythmic	17
Non-cardiac	14
Unwitnessed sudden death	4
Unknown	7

Table 8. Shock and antitachycardia pacing (ATP) episodes

Number of patients	Shock category			Antitachycardia pacing		
	A	I	U	A	I	U
66	422	–	–			
32	–	190	–			
111	–	–	957			
12				210	–	–
4				–	17	–
6				–	–	426

A = appropriate, I = inappropriate, U = unknown; see the text for definitions.

attempted in 15 patients. It was successful in nine. All but one are alive, including the world's very first patient with a non-thoracotomy Endotak system implant [12]. He recently underwent replacement of his subcutaneous defibrillating patch lead secondary to fatigue fracture of the lead at 49 mth post-implant. The single mortality in this group was an in-hospital arrhythmic death following explantation of an infected Endotak AICD.

In our series of 218 patients, three patients have undergone four generator replacements, seven patients three generator replacements, 29 patients two generator replacements, and 51 patients one generator replacement. The remainder of the patients have their original generator implant.

Discussion

After a decade of implantation, the ICD has established itself as a viable and effective therapy for malignant ventricular arrhythmia. Newer devices that have antitachycardia pacing capabilities, such as Cadence V100, have made it possible to terminate some arrhythmic episodes without the need to deliver a DC shock. This type of device, in turn, has expanded the pool of the patients that might benefit from an ICD.

The patients' survival in our series (61% actual survival at 5 yr) parallels that of other major series of patients with ICDs [9,10,13]. Most deaths in the follow-up period were related to deteriorating cardiac function.

A new category of patients who may benefit from ICD is those cardiac transplant candidates with very low left ventricular ejection fraction and apparent high risk for sudden cardiac death. Implantation of an ICD enables these patients to remain more safely in an out-of-hospital environment while awaiting a donor heart. The two instances of infection in ten such patients in our series is disturbing, however. One patient died as a direct result of ICD infection, and in the other an arrhythmic death occurred after the infected system was explanted. Extra precautions are warranted in applying the ICD prophylactically to patients such as these who may already be immunosuppressed from chronic illness and thereby more vulnerable to infection.

A number of complications can occur with these devices. Some are device specific (lead fracture, inappropriate shocks, vascular erosion [10,11,14], constrictive pericarditis [15]) and others are related to the surgical procedure (lung herniations, pleural effusions, atelectasis, etc.). Infection in or around the device is the most devastating complication and can happen in up to 7% of the patients [9,16,17]. The 5.5% incidence of infection in complete ICD systems is within the range of reported infection for these devices, but we feel is unacceptable. We have largely abandoned staged implantation, where leads alone became infected in six of 29 patients (20.7%). Infections have been found to manifest as late as 3 yr following device implantation. The majority of these infections are caused by the slow-growing, slime-producing *Staphylococcus epidermidis* and *Staphylococcus aureus* [9,16]. We believe that appropriate treatment entails the removal of the device in its entirety and implantation of a second system at a later date after all wounds are totally healed. These devices are large and bulky and are constantly at risk of infection, as evidenced by one of our patients who developed infection 29 mth post-implantation. We would recommend that, similar to patients with other types of implants such as prosthetic heart valves, patients with ICDs be treated with appropriate prophylactic antibiotics during any dental or other surgical procedures. Adherence to strict aseptic techniques and attention to minor details during initial implantation, generator change, and lead revision are of utmost importance in minimizing the infectious complications. Currently in our laboratory, we are working with antibiotic binding to the defibrillator patch leads in an attempt to make the AICD more resistant to bacterial seeding.

Fracture of implanted leads, especially the sensing leads, is not infrequent. Winkle et al. [9] reported two instances of sensing lead fracture in 270 patients. We encountered a higher incidence of sensing lead fracture (Table 6). All but one were sutureless screw-in epicardial leads.

With further improvement in technology, the non-thoracotomy implant may become more reliable and gain more acceptance. This, in conjunction with further miniaturization of devices, could make the device more acceptable to the patients and their physicians. Ultimately, this device may be used as a prophylactic measure to prevent sudden cardiac death in those individuals who have a high clinical profile for developing VT and/or VF [12].

References

1. Baum RS, Alvarez HA, Cobb LA (1974) Circulation 50: 1231–1235.
2. Eisenberg MS, Hallstrom A, Bergner L (1982) N Engl J Med 306: 1340–1343.
3. Myerburg RJ, Conde CA, Sung RJ, et al. (1980) Am J Med 68: 568–576.
4. Weaver WD, Lorch GS, Alvarez HA, Cobb LA (1976) Circulation 54: 895–900.
5. Liberthson PR, Nagel EL, Hirschman JC, Nussenfeld SR (1974) N Engl J Med 291: 317–321.
6. Myerburg RJ, Kessler KM, Estes D, et al. (1984) Circulation 70: 538–546.
7. Cobb LA, Werner JA, Trobaugh GB (1980) Modern Concepts Cardiovasc Dis 49: 37–42.
8. Manolis AS, Tan-DeGuzman W, Lee MA, Rastegar H, Haffajee CI, Huang SKS, Estes NAM III (1989) Am Heart J 118: 445–450.
9. Winkle RA, Mead RH, Ruder MA, Gaudiani VA, Smith NA, Buch WS, Schmidt P, Shipman T (1989) J Am Coll Cardiol 13: 1353–1361.
10. Hargrove WC, Josephson ME, Marchlinski FE, Miller JM (1989) J Thorac Cardiovasc Surg 97: 923–928.
11. Olinger GN, Chapman PD, Troup PJ, Almassi GH (1988) J Thorac Cardiovasc Surg 96: 141–149.
12. Troup PJ (1989) Curr Probl Cardiol 14(12).
13. Echt DS, Armstrong K, Schmidt P, Oyer PE, Stinson EB, Winkle RA (1985) Circulation 71: 289–296.
14. Marchlinski FE, Flores BT, Buxton AE, Hargrove WC III, Addonizio VP, Stephenson LW, Harken AH, Doherty JU, Grogan EW Jr, Josephson ME (1986) Ann Intern Med 104: 481–488.
15. Almassi GH, Chapman PD, Troup PJ, Wetherbee JN, Olinger GN (1987) Chest 92: 369–371.
16. Almassi GH, Olinger GN, Troup PJ, Chapman PD, Goodman LR (1988) J Thorac Cardiovasc Surg 95: 908–911.

17. Watkins L Jr, Levine J (1990) In: RB Karp, H Laks and AS Wechsler, eds. Advances in Cardiac Surgery. Chicago: Mosby Year Book, 177–189.

Can cytokines predict rejection in lung transplantation?

Yuichi Yoshida, Yuichi Iwaki, Si Pham, James H. Dauber, Samuel A. Yousem, Adriana Zeevi, Shigeki Morita, Yoshiaki Kita, Kazunori Noguchi, Atsuhito Yagihashi and Bartley P. Griffith

Departments of Pathology and Surgery, University of Pittsburgh School of Medicine, Pittsburgh, PA 15213, U.S.A.

Introduction

Unlike kidney or liver transplant rejection indicators, there are no adequate plasma or serum parameters to diagnose rejection in lung transplantation. As lung transplantation becomes more common, it becomes increasingly important to have some indicators to suggest the presence of rejection.

Cytokines play a critical role in mediating biological responses, particularly in self-defense systems. Interleukin-1β (IL-1β) is released by antigen presentation cells (APC) during the early recognition period of foreign antigen, and Interleukin-2 (IL-2) is released primarily by activated T-lymphocytes following APC presentation [1,2]. Interleukin-6 (IL-6) and tumor necrosis factor α (TNFα) are released by activated macrophages which mediate various biological responses [3–6].

We conducted a study to monitor various cytokines (IL-1β, IL-2, IL-6 and TNFα) in the sera of lung transplant recipients to evaluate whether or not serum cytokine(s) reflect recipients' immune responses.

Materials and Methods

Patient selection

The subjects of this study were five patients undergoing either single lung transplantation (3 patients) or double lung transplantation (2 patients), between November 1990 and December 1990, at Presbyterian University Hospital, University of Pittsburgh.

All patients received similar perioperative intensive care and were immunosuppressed with a combination of cyclosporine A, RATG, steroid and azathioprine.

A histopathological diagnosis was made according to the working formulation for classification and grading of pulmonary rejection [7].

IL-1β, IL-2, IL-6 and TNFα testing

Blood was collected in 5 ml tubes. Serum was immediately obtained and aliquots were stored in polypropylene tubes at −70°C until testing. The daily samples were collected for up to 3 wk unless there was any specific reason to discontinue testing.

Testing for IL-1β, IL-2, IL-6 and TNFα was performed by the 2-step sandwich enzyme immunoassay method using a commercially available ELISA Kit (R&D System Inc., Minneapolis, MN).

Briefly, either 50 μl (IL-1β, IL-6, TNFα) or 200 μl (IL-2) of assay buffer (buffered protein base) were added to 96-well microplates coated with mouse anti-human IL-1β or other monoclonal antibodies (first antibody). Then 200 μl (IL-1β, IL-6, TNFα) or 50 μl (IL-2) of sera were added to microplates. After 2 h incubation at room temperature (IL-1β, IL-2, IL-6) or at 37°C (TNFα) the wells were washed and 200 μl of horseradish peroxidase conjugated goat anti-human IL-1β or other polyclonal antibodies were added. Following an additional 2 h incubation at room temperature, the wells were washed again and incubated at room temperature for 20 min with chromogen (a mixture of H_2O_2 and tetramethylbenzidine). Then, 50 μl of 2 N H_2SO_4 were added to stop the reaction and optical density at 450 nm was measured using a microtiter reader, and serum cytokine levels were obtained from the standard curve. Assay sensitivity was 10 pg/ml.

Results

The serum IL-1β, IL-2, IL-6 or TNFα was not notable in patient F.A., although there were minor fluctuations (Fig. 1). He did not have any significant clinical complications during the monitoring period.

In patient B.H., the peak of serum IL-6 was noted beginning on the 17th post-transplant (PTx) day; however IL-1β, IL-2 and TNFα remained negative (Fig. 2). His post-transplant course was smooth.

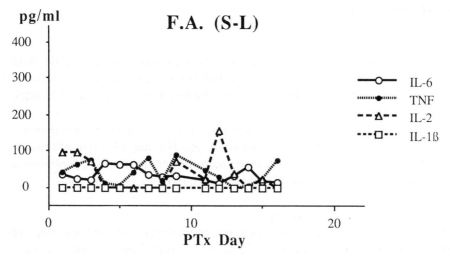

Fig. 1. Serum IL-1β, IL-2, IL-6 and TNFα in patient F.A.

A sharp spike of IL-6 was noted in patient M.M. at the 15th PTx day, but there was no elevation of IL-1β and TNFα (Fig. 3). Similarly, a spike of serum IL-2 was observed during the same period. The biopsy-confirmed acute cellular rejection was coincidentally observed 2 days after IL-6 and IL-2 elevation.

A consistently high level of serum IL-6 was noted in patient P.S. (Fig. 4). In addition, her serum TNFα level had 2 demonstrable peaks. Two days after the first peak, the biopsy-proven acute cellular rejection was observed. The decrease in her serum TNFα coincided with the 3-day bolus steroid therapy. IL-1β and IL-2 remained within the normal limit. She had repeated episodes of bronchitis with

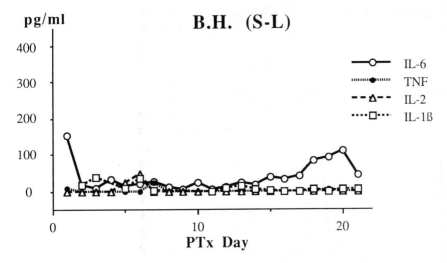

Fig. 2. Serum IL-1β, IL-2, IL-6 and TNFα in patient B.H.

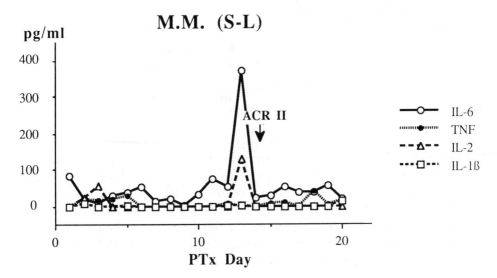

Fig. 3. Serum IL-1β, IL-2, IL-6 and TNFα in patient M.M.

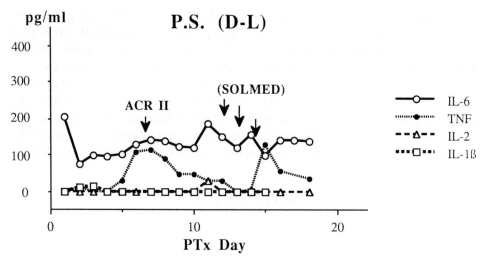

Fig. 4. Serum IL-1β, IL-2, IL-6 and TNFα in patient P.S.

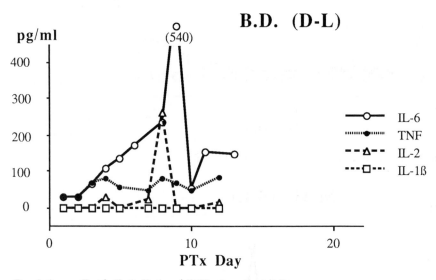

Fig. 5. Serum IL-1β, IL-2, IL-6 and TNFα in patient B.D.

concomitant CMV infection, which was probably transmitted by the donor.

Patient B.D. suffered from the preservation injury combined with pneumonia. The serum IL-6 level started to increase on the 4th PTx day and remained at a high level (Fig. 5). A sharp spike of IL-2 was observed on the 8th PTx day, and a sharp spike of IL-6 was observed on the 9th PTx day. Although the serum TNFα remained moderately high throughout the course, IL-1β did not increase. A biopsy was not performed.

Discussion

Although the number of patients in this study was limited, of the four cytokines that we examined serum IL-6 appears to furnish some clinical significance in single- or double-lung transplantation. IL-6 is produced by activated T-lymphocytes, macrophages and endothelial cells as well as fibroblasts [3,4]. IL-6 production seems to be more significant in lung transplantation compared to other solid organ transplantation, probably because of the presence of alveolar macrophages. In fact, there was a clear spike of IL-6 in patient M.M. 2 days prior to the biopsy-proven acute cellular rejection. Similarly, patient B.H. had an IL-6 spike although a histopathological study was not performed.

IL-6 is also produced in the presence of systemic infection [8]. Patient P.S. had repeated bronchitis with concomitant CMV infection. Her serum IL-6 level was consistently high. Interestingly, she demonstrated two dull elevated slopes of IL-6, which coincided with the presence of rejection. Furthermore, serum TNFα in this patient seemed to correlate with the presence of rejection, indicating that a combination of IL-6 and TNFα could be useful.

In patients F.A. and M.M., minor spikes of serum IL-2 were noted. It seems that they might be associated with the presence of rejections; however, it was too premature to form a conclusion. Further studies are required.

Serum IL-1β was not demonstrated in this study. It is possible that the biological activity of IL-1β is too short to be assayed; however, the possibility that our assay system was not sensitive should not be overlooked.

In summary, of the four cytokines, IL-6 seems to be a useful marker for a lung transplant patient because its sharp spike is associated with the presence of rejection and its persistent elevation indicates the presence of infection.

Acknowledgement

This study was supported in part by a grant from the University of Pittsburgh Pathology Education and Research Foundation.

References

1. Maury CPJ, Teppo AM (1990) Serum immunoreactive interleukin-1 in renal transplant recipients. Transplantation 49: 1070.
2. Cantrell DA, Smith KA (1984) The Interleukine-2, T cell system. A new cell growth factor. Science 224: 1312.
3. Kishimoto T (1989) The biology of Interleukin-6. Blood 74: 10.
4. Van Snick J (1990) Interleukin-6: an overview. Annu Rev Immunol 8: 253.
5. Economou JS, NcBride WH, Essner R, et al. (1989) Tumor necrosis factor production by interleukin-2 activated macrophages in vitro and in vivo. Immunology 67: 514.
6. Imagawa DK, Millis JM, Olthoff KM, et al (1990) The role of tumor necrosis factor in allograft rejection. Transplantation 50: 219.

7. Yousem SA, Berry GJ, Brunt EM, et al. (1990) A working formulation for the Standardization of Nomenclature in the Diagnosis of Heart and Lung Rejection: Lung Rejection Study Group. J Heart Transplant 9: 593.

8. Hack CE, De Groot ER, Felt-Bersam JFF, et al. (1989) Increased plasma levels of interleukin-6 in sepsis. Blood 74: 1704.

Development and clinical experience of a new tabletop cardiopulmonary bypass system for percutaneous cardiopulmonary support and extracorporeal membrane oxygenation

Y. Sasako[1], T. Nakatani[2], H. Akagi[2], Y. Baba[2], Y. Taenaka[2], H. Takano[2], K. Nishigaki[1], H. Doi[1], Y. Kito[1] and Y. Kawashima[1]

[1]Department of Cardiovascular Surgery and [2]Research Institute, National Cardiovascular Center, Suita, Osaka, 565, Japan

Introduction

Cardiopulmonary bypass (CPB) techniques have been used for circulatory support cardiac resuscitation, and respiratory support. Recently, it has begun to be used as an assisting procedure during percutaneous transluminal coronary angioplasty (PTCA). However, it takes much time and considerable amount of priming volume to set up the usual CPB system. In order to solve these problems, we have developed a new tabletop CPB system with quick assembly and small priming volume. This new system was applied to extracorporeal membrane oxygenation (ECMO), supported PTCA and percutaneous cardiopulmonary support (PCPS).

A new tabletop CPB system

The circuit of the new system consists of two parts. One is a sterile package containing arterial and venous tubes with a filter in between. The other is an unsterile portion with a centrifugal pump, a membrane oxygenator and a priming port (Fig. 1). No reservoir or heat exchanger is installed. The filter (Pole, ECP-3 LPM) accelerates deaeration on priming, so the system can be primed and be prepared on the table within 5 min (even 3 min with the newest model).

The notable efficacy of this system comes from a newly developed membrane oxygenator (Kuraray, Menox EL-4000 / 2000). It achieved the reduction of priming volume and the downsizing of the system itself. Also its long-term stable function solved the problem of frequent renewals of the oxygenator. Priming volume of the system is as low as 500 ml (adult PCPS with filter), 250 ml (adult ECMO) or 200 ml (pediatric ECMO).

In the first model of this system, Biopump (Biomedicus, BP-80 or 50) was installed. In the recent model, Sarns Delphin Pump is used for easier deaeration. The system shown in Fig. 1 is a prototype model, and a smaller package for emergent PCPS and supported PTCA is being developed.

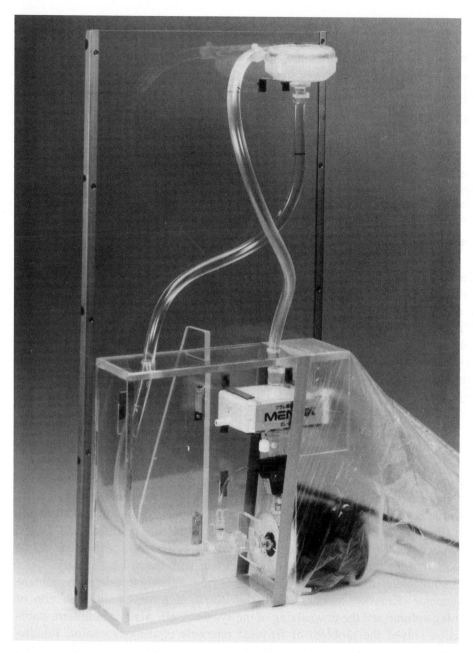

Fig. 1. New tabletop CPB system.

A newly developed membrane oxygenator

This oxygenator has several prominent features as follows: (1) an ultra compact size with a low priming volume (EL-4000: max flow 4 l/min, membrane surface area 0.8 m^2, priming volume 110 ml; EL-2000: 2 l/min, 0.4 m^2, 50 ml); (2) a high gas exchange performance with an efficient disposition of hollow fibers (Fig. 2); (3) a novel gas exchange membrane made of polyolefin in which micropores are blind at the blood contacting surface to prevent serum leakage (Fig. 3).

Clinical experiences

This system was clinically used for five adult and three pediatric cases. Indications included respiratory failure (RF) in 4, supported PTCA in 2 cases, cardiogenic shock in 1, and intractable ventricular tachycardia (VT) following acute myocardial infarction (AMI) in 1 (Table 1). Duration of support was from 2 h of supported PTCA to 12 days of respiratory support. No renewal of membrane oxygenator was done for the deterioration of its performance. This system was useful in pediatric ECMO because of low hemodilution and easy maintenance with few renewals. In one of the ECMO cases (case 2, Fig. 4), the

Table 1. Clinical Cases.

Cases	Age	Sex	Diagnosis	Indication	Type	Flow (l/min)	Effect	Result	Duration
Case 1	6 mth	f	CAVC, Post op.	Respiratory support	V-V V-A	0.2	fair	CHF	4 d
Case 2	1 mth	f	TGA, Post op.	Respiratory support	V-A	1.0	good	CHF	12 d
Case 3	6 yr	f	Thoraco-esophageal fistel	Respiratory support during op.	V-V	1.0	good	Fistelec-tomy	8 h
Case 4	48 yr	f	ECD, PMI, shock CHF(on VAS)	Respiratory support	V-A	2.0	good	LV rupture	6 h
Case 5	54 yr	m	AP, CHF, OMI, equivalent LMT	Supported PTCA	V-A	4.0	good	PTCA	2 h
Case 6	58 yr	f	AP, equivalent LMT	Supported PTCA	V-A	3.0	good	PTCA	2 h
Case 7	53 yr	m	CAD, Post CABG PMI, shock	Circulatory support	V-A	5.0	good	re CABG	6 h
Case 8	53 yr	m	AMI, VT, CHF	Vt unloading	V-A	3.0	good	cryosurgery	2 d

CAD, coronary artery disease; CABG, coronary artery bypass grafting; PMI, perioperative myocardial infarction; AMI, acute myocardial infarction; VT, intractable ventricular tachycardia; CHF, congestive heart failure; AP, angina pectoris; LMT, left main trunc lesion; OMI, old myocardial infarction; ECD, endocardial cushion defect; VAS, ventricular assist system; TGA, transposition of great arteries; CAVC, complete atrio-ventricular cannal; PTCA, percutaneous transluminal coronary angioplasty; V-A, veno-arterial bypass; V-V, veno-venous bypass.

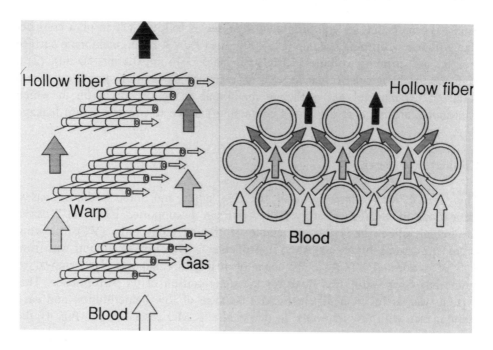

Fig. 2. Structure of the newly developed membrane oxygenator; an efficient disposition of hollow fibers produces a high gas exchange performance.

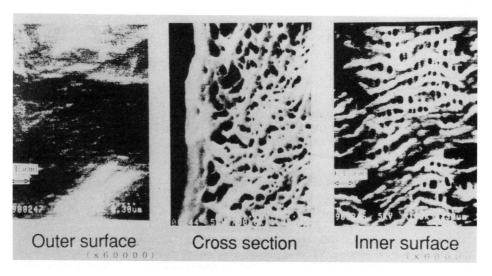

Fig. 3. A novel gas exchange membrane made of polyolefin. Micropores are blind at the blood-contacting surface to prevent serum leakage.

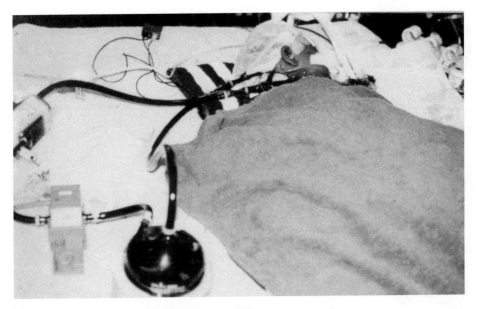

Fig. 4. Tabletop CPB system in a pediatric ECMO.

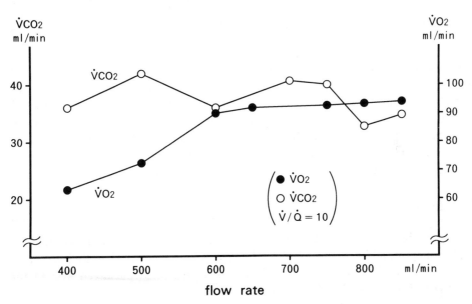

Fig. 5. Oxygen transfer rate ($\dot{V}O_2$) and carbon dioxide removal rate ($\dot{V}CO_2$) in a pediatric ECMO after continuous usage for 1 wk.

gas exchange performance of this oxygenator (EL-2000) was studied with her parents' permission. Despite its compact size and usage for one week, oxygen transfer rate (VO_2) and carbon dioxide removal rate (VCO_2) of this oxygenator were 90 ml/min and 35 ml/min, respectively (Fig. 5). In 2 supported PTCA cases,

194

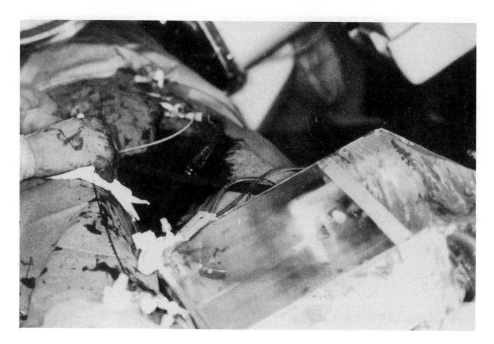

Fig. 6. Tabletop CPB system during supported PTCA.

this system was safely and easily mobilized, being placed on the patient's bed during catheterization (Fig. 6). In a case of cardiogenic shock, operation was performed with this system (case 7). In case 8, no attack of VT occurred for 2 days during support. This system proved to be effective in all 8 cases. Perfusion flow rate ranged between 2.0 and 5.0 l/min in adult cases. Blood hemoglobin concentration and body temperature of the patients were stable during the process of CPB using this system. There were no complications related to this system.

Conclusion

Based on these results, we conclude that our tabletop CPB system is suitable for PCPS, supported PTCA and ECMO. The downsizing and easy handling to set up brought no adverse effect. Our final goal is a preprimed packaged system for quicker and easier application to emergency cases.

References

1. Hirose H, Matsuda H, Kawashima Y (1984) Mechanical control of circulation; clinical results with intra-arotic balloon pumping and veno-arterial bypass in left and/or right cardiogenic failure. Jpn Circ J 48: 288-294.
2. Kennedy JH (1969) Assisted circulation: an extended concept of cardiopulmonary resuscitation. J Thorac Cardiovasc Surg 57: 688-701.

3. Blale LH (1976) Goals and progress of the National Heart and Lung Institute collaborative extracorporeal membrane oxygenation study. Artificial lungs for acute respiratory failure. Washington DC: Hemisphere, 297.

4. Vogel RA, Shawl F, et al. (1990) Initial report of the national Registry of elective cardiopulmonary bypass supported coronary angioplasty. J Am Coll Cardiol 15: 23-29.

5. Reichmann RT, Joyo CI, Dembitsky WP, et al. (1990) Improved patient survival after cardiac arrest using a cardio-pulmonary support system. Ann Thorac Surg 49: 101-105.

6. Tatsumi E, Takenaka Y, Nakatani T, et al. (1991) A VAD and novel high performance compact oxygenator for long-term ECMO with local anticoagulation. ASAIO Trans 36: M480-483.

7. Doi H, Sasako Y, Tatsumi E, et al. (1991) A case report of extracorporeal membrane oxygenation in infant using KURARAY 'KMO' membrane oxygenator. Jpn J Artif Organs 20: 1114-1117.

Ventricular assist device as a mechanical support for postcardiotomy failure and as a bridge to heart transplantation

M. Shiono, G.P. Noon and Y. Nosé

Department of Surgery, Baylor College of Medicine, One Baylor Plaza, Houston, TX 77030, U.S.A.

Introduction

Mechanical circulatory support has been successfully used and considerable experience has been obtained in patients with ventricular failure. Ventricular assist devices (VADs) and total artificial hearts (TAHs) have demonstrated clinical capabilities of far more profound circulatory support with the potential of increasing use during recent years. These devices have also been employed to support a small number of hemodynamically deteriorating transplant candidates until a suitable donor heart has been obtained. These experiences have made a dramatic impact on specific patients with dismal prognosis. As of December 1990, these devices have been applied in more than 1400 patients with heart failure according to the report in the International Registry [1]. In this paper, we review and describe several devices that have been used clinically and discuss the results.

Mechanical circulatory support

All support devices have been used as the alternative when the patient becomes refractory to conventional treatments. These methods are classified into three categories; series assist, parallel assist and replacement [2].

Series assist devices use the entire left ventricular output ejected to the aorta and are used as a counterpulsation device, such as IABP. Hemopump (Johnson & Johnson) has a unique feature and is classified as an axial flow pump [3]. This intraaortic device can generate 3 l/min of flow and decompresses the failing left ventricle without applying counterpulsation. Flow rate is dependent on the afterload of the systemic circulation. This type of axial flow pump is promising in more profound heart failure populations beyond IABP.

Parallel assist devices include several systems that have been recently applied in many patients and called VAD [4–6]. VAD is placed in parallel with the native ventricle and drains the blood from the atrium or the ventricle and returns it to the arteries. The device decompresses the ventricle and assists the systemic or pulmonary circulation by generating 3–10 l/min of blood flow. These devices are divided into three categories according to their assist method: left ventricular assist devices (LVADs), right ventricular assist devices (RVADs) and combined biventricular assist devices (BVADs). Currently available pusatile devices are pneumatic systems and electrical systems, according to their driving source (Table 1).

These devices have a pump and cannulae. The draining cannula is inserted into the left atrium or left ventricle and the perfusion cannula into the aorta in an LVAD. Right atrium and pulmonary artery are used for inflow and outflow respectively in RVADs. There are several options for positioning and placing the cannulae and pump (Fig. 1).

Table 1. Available VADs

Source	Mode	Name	Assist Period	Position
Pneumatic		Thoratec, Abiomed	short or intermediate	para-, extra-corporeal
		Zeon, Toyobo, Berlin	short or intermediate	para-, extra-corporeal
		TCI	intermediate or long	abdominal cavity
Electrical	Pulsatile	Novacor	intermediate or long	intra-abdominal wall
		CCF	intermediate or long	intra-thoracic
	Nonpulsatile	Roller pump	short	extra-corporeal
		Centrifugal;	short	extra-corporeal
		Biomedicus, Sarns		

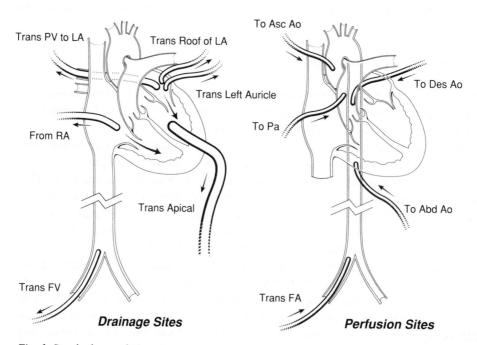

Drainage Sites

Perfusion Sites

Fig. 1. Standard cannulation sites.

Left ventricular cannulation requires cardiopulmonary bypass. With Novacor (Baxter) and TCI (Thermo-Cardiac systems) devices, the draining cannula has to be inserted into left ventricular apex for adequate pump flow under bypass. The Thoratec pump (3M) has several options for draining cannulae.

Several devices of different sizes, shapes and power sources have developed to maintain both systemic and pulmonary circulation without native ventricles as in *mechanical replacement* [7]. All TAHs applied clinically are pneumatically driven systems and the patients are linked to the external driving console. The Jarvik-7 TAH (Symbion) has been the most frequently used device and contributed to a new field of clinical practice as a bridge-to-heart transplantation [8].

Clinical application

The indications for mechanical assist are (1) postcardiotomy cardiogenic shock, (2) endstage heart failure due to cardiomyopathy, (3) cardiogenic shock due to acute myocardial infarction and (4) miscellaneous.

The indications for support in the postcardiotomy setting have been divided into two categories: the unsuccessful cases of weaning from cardiopulmonary bypass and the cases with low output syndrome after cardiotomy. Postcardiotomy applications have been expected to be approximately 1–2% of all patients undergoing cardiac operations. The indications for support in conjunction with heart transplantation have been divided into three categories; hemodynamic deterioration before transplantation, acute rejection after transplantation, and immediate donor heart failure after transplantation considered not to be related to acute rejection.

Hemodynamic criteria
The hemodynamic criteria for application of the mechanical support [9] have been proposed to be a cardiac index of less than 1.8 l/min/m^2, pulmonary capillary wedge pressure greater than 25 mmHg, and systolic arterial pressure less than 80 mmHg in LVADs despite maximal medical therapy including IABP. The overall clinical impression is added to these parameters as an important criterion. RVAD has been applied or added with a cardiac index of less than 2.0 l/min/m^2 and CVP more than 30 cm H$_2$O despite left ventricular assistance. There have been many additional criteria and modifications in different clinical situations.

Device selection
The diagnosis of left, right or biventricular failure is important in determining what type of device should be used (Table 1). Etiology of the ventricular failure is also important in determining how long mechanical support should be continued. In most cases left ventricular assist is initiated first and this may unmask right ventricular failure, necessitating right ventricular assist. When the patient has severe biventricular failure and has already been selected as a

candidate for heart transplantation, TAHs or BVADs should be applied. When the cardiac function is expected to be reversible, short-term (less than 1 wk) or inter-mediate-term (1 wk to 1 mth) devices, i.e. centrifugal pump, pneumatic VADs, may be indicated. However, currently available devices are limited to use only in a few major institutions. In order to establish the management of profound ventricular failure, these devices should be spread widely.

Results

There continues to be reasonable enthusiasm for the application of the devices, as evidenced by the data from International Registry report, indicating a number of patients supported by these devices during the last several years. In this report, clinically applied devices are divided into two categories; i.e. postcardiotomy support and bridge-to-transplantation.

Postcardiotomy support

While VADs could salvage patients who would have died without mechanical support, the overall results in the postcardiotomy setting has been discouraging. As of December 1990, VADs have been used in 965 patients for postcardiotomy support. The weaning rate from the device is 45% and the mean survival rate is 25% (discharged). 67% of all patients have been supported by centrifugal devices and this is expected to be due to limited availability of pulsatile devices. There are not statistical differences of survival rate between centrifugal and pneumatic devices. Average assist period is approximately 4 days in LVAD, RVAD and BVAD. When BVADs are required, survival rate reflects the severity of the ventricular failure and is diminished compared to LVADs or RVADs (20%, 28% and 26% respectively) (Table 2).

Bridge-to-transplantation

Mechanical assist has been employed to support deteriorating transplant candidates until a suitable donor heart has been obtained: 'bridge to trans-plantation' [10]. The most substantial development of treatment has been the application of mechanical support in this population. The early results are

Table 2. VADs in postcardiotomy cardiogenic shock

VAD	Cases	Weaned	Discharged
LVAD	494	254 (51%)	137 (28%)
RVAD	121	47 (39%)	31 (26%)
BVAD	350	132 (38%)	69 (20%)
Total	965	433 (45%)	237 (25%)

Data from ASAIO-ISHT Registry.

encouraging and have made a dramatic impact on this new field. As of December 1990, VADs and TAHs have been used in 476 patients for bridge-to-trans- plantation. 69% of the patients who have been supported by these devices have been transplanted and the mean survival rate is 66% in transplanted cases. Of 476 patients overall who received mechanical assist, 26% received LVADs, 34% received BVADs and 40% received TAHs. Univentricular RVADs are rarely indicated in this setting. The rates of subsequent transplantation are similar regardless of type of support used: 71% for LVADs, 65% BVADs, and 71% TAHs. The discharge rate is significantly different among these groups: 87% for LVADs, 70% BVADs, and 50% TAHs (Table 3).

Patients with univentricular LVADs approach the same actuarial survival rate as with the standard transplant. These results have been due to satisfactory results contributed by long-term (more than 1 mth) devices. Average assist period is approximately 31 days in LVADs, 20 days in RVADs, 15 days in BVADs and 24 days in TAHs.

Complications
Complications are frequent in this critically ill group of patients [11]. Bleeding is the most common complication, occurring in 30–40% of all patients. Renal

Table 3. VADs and TAHs in staged transplantation

VAD/TAH	Cases	Transplanted	Discharged
LVAD	122	87 (71%)	76 (87%)
RVAD	4	1 (25%)	1 (100%)
BVAD	161	105 (65%)	73 (70%)
TAH	189	135 (71%)	67 (50%)
Total	476	328 (68%)	217 (66%)

Data from ASAIO-ISHT Registry.

Table 4. Major complications during postcardiotomy VADs

Complication	Incidence	
	Weaned cases (%)	Not weaned cases (%)
Bleeding/DIC	49	41
Renal failure	36	26
Biventricular failure	34	16
Cannula obstruction/low cardiac output	21	9
Infection	7	19
Thromboembolism	9	12

Data from ASAIO-ISHT Registry.

Table 5. Major complications associated with mechanical assistance in bridge use

Complication	VAD (%) (n = 38)	BVAD (%) (n = 56)	TAH (%) (n = 54)
Bleeding	31	25	27
Biventricular failure	45	43	0
Renal failure	31	27	40
Respiratory failure	17	18	42
Infection	21	14	36
MOF	0	11	29

Data from ASAIO-ISHT Registry. * Precluding transplantation. MOF, multiple organ failure.

failure, infection, poor cardiac output are also the major complications encountered (Tables 4 and 5).

Discussion

In clinical applications of the devices, there have been many problems that have been encountered and should be solved. Patient selection and timing of the implantation are the most critical problem. In cases where mechanical assists has been applied, poor preoperative cardiac function and latent organ failure progressed to MOF by additional risks of surgical intervention and cardiopulmonary bypass. Any significant life-saving effect of mechanical support has still been poor. During mechanical assist, total cardiac output index is maintained at 2.2–2.5 $l/min/m^2$ because a low output state already complicates recovery from the latent injuries to the vital organs. An early application is essential for obtaining a better result.

Selection of the appropriate device and implantation technique are important factors to consider. Centrifugal and external pulsatile device can be used for left ventricular support with or without right support, and can be used in either the atria or the left ventricle. In postcardiotomy or postinfarction cardiogenic shock, left atrial cannulation is preferable because it avoids additional damage to the myocardium. In potential transplant candidates, left ventricular cannulation is preferred in order to obtain a sufficient pump flow. The position of the pump and cannulae should be considered with careful attention for obtaining better hemodynamics and avoiding complications, i.e. bleeding and infection. The results in the bridge-to-transplant population have been contributed by the use of intermediate-term or long-term devices. As the number of heart transplantations has increased so has the waiting time for obtaining a suitable heart. The long-term devices, such as Novacor (Baxter) and TCI (Thermo-Cardiac systems) devices, have been applied for this specific population. The LVAD developed at Cleveland Clinic (CCF) has been implanted successfully for more than 5 mth.

Recent results of TCI implantation in 11 cases supported over a 30-day period as a bridge-to-transplant device have demonstrated a 100% survival rate after transplantation (Frazier OH, personal communication). However, clinical applications of these devices are restricted by the Food and Drug Administration as IDE (Investigational Device Exemption) in the United States. At the present time, availability of the devices is limited and only a few institutions have permission to implant a certain device. Thoratec pump, Novacor and TCI devices have not been widely available. This leaves heart bypass or conventional ventricular assist with short-term devices, such as BioMedicus or Sarns centrifugal pump, as the only method of support. Abroad, there have already been some commercially available devices, such as Nippon Zeon VAD, Toyobo VAD (Japan) and Berlin Assist Heart (Germany). Implantable LVADs have not been commercially available. Another problem is that the implantable devices have not been efficient in severe biventricular failure and a TAH would be necessary as a replacement device for intermediate-term or long-term assistance.

In the pre-, intra- and post-device patient care, special care should be taken to maintain the other vital organ functions that affect the prognosis of patients in optimal condition. An anticoagulation regimen has been one of the essential treatments and almost all patients have received some type of anticoagulant during support. However, a uniform anticoagulation regimen has not been defined for any of the devices. At present, all the devices need some anticoagulant therapy to avoid thromboembolism. Bleeding is another major complication and sometimes related to coagulopathy. To prevent this complication careful attention should be paid to the implant procedure, anticoagulant therapy and monitoring of the coagulation system. Infectious complications are common during and after mechanical support. This complication is expected to be relevant to multiple organ failure in these critically ill patients. Device-centered infection is an important problem, especially in TAHs. It is understood that the implantation of a device in the mediastinum (Jarvik-7) is not clinically feasible whereas the devices implanted inside either the abdominal cavity or abdominal wall are acceptable without causing infection. However, it is necessary to consider all the possible causes for the higher infection rate of Jarvik-7 TAH [12]. Prophylaxis is the only way of avoiding this complication and it seems to be a principal factor to maintain the patient in optimal condition.

At present, none of the devices mentioned here can be relied on to function without a possibility of thromboembolism. Many devices have been using polyurethanes as antithrombogenic material and it is also expected that biolization or endothelialization will be available as blood-contacting surface in the future. In the engineering problem, consideration should be given not only to antithrombogenicity but also to the improvement of the pump, cannula, connection parts, prosthetic valve, and the size and flow rate of the pump. Continuous development and modifications are expected in the various parts of the devices.

As to the socioeconomic problems, it has been obvious that intensive care for patients with circulatory support is quite expensive, especially in long-term periods. How do we treat the patients who cannot beweaned from assist devices with MOF? It has been also argued that mechanical assistance cannot increase the number of transplants in the limited situation of donor heart availability. Are more stable candidates excluded from transplant if supported patients have priority? Is the implantable long-term VAD really cost-effective? There are many arguments and problems that should be solved socially, economically and ethically.

Conclusion

A number of patients with mechanical circulatory support have accumulated in the last several years and a new clinical field of bridge-to-transplantation has been introduced in the last decade. A variety of devices for circulatory support are under development. However, most of these devices are not clinically available. It is hoped that these devices will be simple to implant, cost-effective and widely available in the near future. After careful analysis of the results in the accumulated patient population, many problems encountered in the past might be resolved in the future. Continued efforts are required to improve further the medical, engineering and the socioeconomical problems in accordance with the advances in ventricular assist devices.

References

1. ASAIO-ISHT: combined registry report (1991) Pennsylvania State University.
2. Ghosh PK (1989) In: F Unger, ed. Assisted Circulation 3. Berlin: Springer-Verlag, 8–45.
3. Frazier OH, Macris MP, Wampler RK, et al. (1990) J Heart Transplant 9: 408–414.
4. Magovern GJ, Park SB, Maher TD (1985) World J Surg 9: 25–36.
5. Pennington DG, Kanter KR, McBride LR, et al. (1988) J Thorac Cardiovasc Surg 96: 901–911.
6. Portner PM, Oyer PE, Pennington DG, et al. (1989) Ann Thorac Surg 47: 142–150.
7. Unger F, et al. (1989) In: F Unger, ed. Assisted Circulation 3. Berlin: Springer-Verlag, 329–419.
8. Joyce LD, Johnson KE, Pierce WS, et al. (1986) J Heart Transplant 5: 229–235.
9. Pierce WS, Parr GVS, Myers JL, et al. (1981) N Engl J Med 305: 1606–1610.
10. Magovern JA, Pierce WS (1990) In: WA Baumgartner, ed. Heart Transplantation. Philadelphia: Saunders, 73–85.
11. Kriett JM, Kaye MP (1990) J Heart Transplant 9: 323–330.
12. Nosé Y (1991) Artif Organs 15: 161–163.

Cardio-thoracic surgery. K. Minami et al. editors.

Follow-up clinical status up to 6 years after multivessel angioplasty with regard to the degree of revascularization

H. Seggewiß[1], D. Faßbender[1], J. Vogt[1], H.K. Schmidt[1], K. Minami[2] and U. Gleichmann[1]

[1]Department of Cardiology, [2]Department of Thoracic and Cardiovascular Surgery, Heart Center Nordrhein Westfalen, Ruhr – University Bochum, 4970 Bad Oeynhausen, F.R.G.

Introduction

Percutaneous transluminal coronary angioplasty (PTCA) has become established in the therapy of patients with single vessel coronary artery disease (CAD) only a few years after its introduction by Grüntzig in 1977 [1]. Multivessel (MV) PTCA increasingly gains clinical importance although its efficacy has not been proved by randomized trials [2-6,8,9]. It will take some time before the results of the different ongoing randomized studies (GABI, RITA, BARI, CABRI, EAST) are available [10]. Therefore, cardiologists have to make their clinical decisions in patients with multivessel disease on the basis of nonrandomized retrospective or prospective trials. These investigations take a particular interest in the clinical outcome of patients with complete revascularization in comparison to patients with incomplete revascularization [3,6,7,9]. In this study we present the acute results and follow-up status of patients who underwent MV PTCA in our institution between January 1985 and July 1989.

Methods

Patient profiles
Between January 1985 and July 1989, 2563 angioplasties were performed in our institution with strict surgical stand-by, given by the Department of Thoracic and Cardiovascular Surgery. 231 patients (9%) underwent MV PTCA, another 115 patients had multilesion PTCA. Six patients where MV PTCA was initially planned were excluded from the study population after failed PTCA of the culprit lesion. Two of them underwent emergency bypass surgery and 4 patients had elective bypass surgery. Clinical and agiographic baseline characteristics of the patients with MV PTCA are listed in Table 1.

Angioplasty procedure
The routinely used premedication, the medication during the angioplasty, and the technical procedure are described elsewhere [11]. In order to minimize the patients' risk and to achieve optimal clinical results we use the following dilatation strategy in patients with MV PTCA. First we recanalize a total

Table 1. Clinical and angiographic characteristics in patients with MV PTCA between I/1985 and VII/1989

Patients (*n*) 231; age (yr) 57 ± 9 (34–78).

	n	%
Men	202	87
Women	29	13
Previous MI	116	50
Non Q-wave	14	6
Q-wave	102	44
Previous PTCA	35	15
Previous CABG	18	8
Clinical indication		
Stable angina	185	81
Unstable angina	17	7
Post MI angina	20	8
Silent ischemia	9	4
Single vessel disease	36	15
Double vessel disease	163	71
Triple vessel disease	32	14
LV - EF < 50%	55	24
LV - EF (%)	69 ± 11	

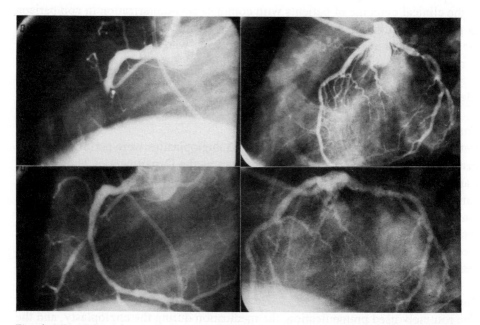

Fig. 1. MV PTCA of a 50-yr-old man with CTO of the RCA (upper panel, left) receiving collaterals by the severely stenotic CX and the LAD (upper panel, right). Final result after recanalization of the RCA (lower panel, left) and PTCA of the CX (lower panel, right).

occlusion supplying ischemic myocardium, especially if it receives collaterals by a stenotic coronary artery, supplying the largest zone of ischemic myocardium, the culprit lesion. Then we dilate other vessels with reference to their technical difficulty – 'worst first'. The strategy is illustrated in Fig. 1. Before and after MV PTCA coronary angiograms were visually analysed by two experienced cardiologists by reviewing at least two orthogonal projections. In order to describe the procedure and the acute and follow-up results the following definitions were used.

Multivessel PTCA Angioplasty of two or more lesions in two or more coronary arteries and/or major side branches – for example the LAD and first diagonal branch.

Multilesion PTCA Angioplasty of two or more lesions in different parts of one coronary artery or a major side branch.

Technical success At least 20% reduction of the initial percent diameter stenosis and postangioplasty diameter stenosis of <50%.

Clinical success Angiographic success in at least the culprit lesion and improvement of cardiac complaints; no major ischemic complications (myocardial infarction, emergency bypass surgery, death) during PTCA.

Complete revascularization No residual stenosis >50% left in any coronary artery or a major side branch after PTCA.

Restenosis Residual stenosis >50% at control angiography.

Cardiac event Evidence of re-PTCA, PTCA of another lesion, bypass surgery (CABG), acute myocardial infarction (AMI), or cardiac death during follow-up.

Follow-up status
Angiographic follow-up was achieved in 181 patients (79%), with 378 dilated lesions (74%), after 3–4 mth. Clinical follow-up status after 31.2 mth to 6 yr could be achieved by questionnaire or telephone interview of the patients or family doctors in all 229 primarily successful treated patients.

Primary results

A total of 508 lesions were dilated; that means 2.2 lesions per patient: 93.1% of all attempted lesions were successfully treated. Initially 229 patients (99.1%) had clinically successful angioplasty: in 198 patients (86%) all attempted stenoses were successfully treated, in 31 patients (13%) dilatation of one of the attempted lesions failed (Table 2). In two further patients angioplasty of two or more

208

lesions failed: the first patient with two type C lesions had successful second dilatation a few days later, the second patient underwent emergency bypass

Table 2. Technical success, clinical success, and degree of revascularization after MV PTCA

	n	%
Lesions	508	100
Technical success	473	93.1
Failure	35	6.9
Patients		
Clinical success	229	99.1
Success all lesions	198	85.7
Failure 1 lesion	31	13.4
Failure	2	0.9
Revascularization		
Complete	164	71.0
Incomplete, second PTCA	11	4.7
Post MI Angina	54	23.4

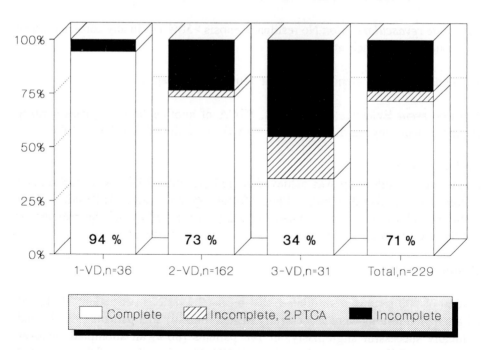

Fig. 2. Degree of revascularization with regard to the extent of coronary artery disease after MV PTCA.

surgery (EBS) because of an early reocclusion of 1 vessel with subsequent cardiogenic shock after initially successful PTCA of 4 lesions. The incidence of EBS was 1.3% in the observed period in consideration of the two patients who had EBS after failed PTCA of the culprit lesion. After MV PTCA 72% of the patients had complete revascularization (Fig. 2).

Follow-up status
Angiographic follow-up was achieved in 181 patients and 378 lesions after 3–4 mth. The incidence of lesion-related restenosis was 29% (2% reocclusion and 27% restenosis) and thus comparable to patients with single lesion angioplasty. The risk of having a restenosis in patients with MV PTCA was 49%; 36% had restenosis of one lesion and 13% had restenoses of two lesions (Fig. 3).

In March 1991 clinical follow-up status was documented in all 229 patients with clinically successful MV PTCA. Mean follow-up period was 31.2 mth (up to 6 yr) without any difference between patients with complete and incomplete revascularization. 223 patients were still alive; 3 patients died for cardiac and noncardiac reasons. Degree of revascularization had no influence on survival (Table 2).

Cardiac events occurred in 34.9% of the patients, with re-PTCA having the largest share with 21.8%. In 4.4% of the patients PTCA of other lesions were done. The incidence of required bypass operations was 6.5% in all patients. Only

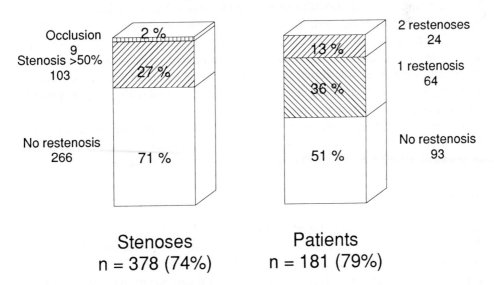

Fig. 3. Angiographic follow-up after MV PTCA.

210

Cardiac Events

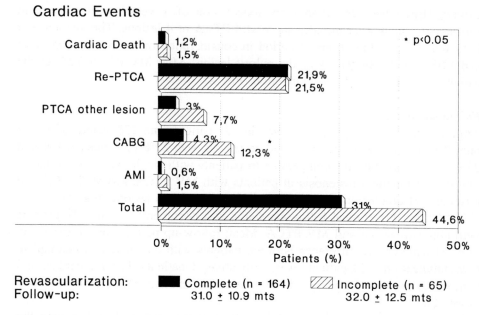

Fig. 4. Cardiac events after MV PTCA with regard to the degree of revascularization.

two patients suffered myocardial infarction during follow-up. The great number of revascularization procedures in our study may be the reason for the low incidence of myocardial infarctions and cardiac deaths during follow-up (Table 2).

If we analyse the incidence of cardiac events with regard to the degree of revascularization we see no difference in the total number of cardiac events (31% compared with 44.6%), cardiac deaths (1.2% compared with 1.5%), re-PTCA (21.9% compared with 21.5%), PTCA of another lesion (3.0% compared with 7.7%), and myocardial infarction (0.6% compared with 1.5%). The only significant difference was found in the incidence of required bypass operations: 4.3% in patients with complete revascularization compared with 12.3% in patients with incomplete revascularization (Fig. 4).

In the 223 living patients cardiac complaints were improved in 79%. Deterioration of angina was observed in 17% of patients (Table 3). The degree of revascularization had no influence on clinical follow-up status.

Discussion

Angioplasty has been established in the therapy of single vessel CAD. Although there was a lack of randomized trials, indication for performing PTCA was widened to patients with MV CAD if the angioplasty could result in nearly complete revascularization [12]. There is a general agreement that MV PTCA can be safely performed in patients with several Type A and Type B lesions [12]. On the other hand the indication for MV PTCA is not given in the presence of several Type C lesions, especially chronic total occlusions >3 mth, serving large amounts of viable myocardium.

PTCA of patients with MV CAD shows an increased risk compared with angioplasty in patients with single vessel CAD [13,14]. In contrast to that, MV PTCA has no increased risk of acute ischemic complications [5,9,14,15]. The reason therefore may be the careful patient selection that gave special attention to the potential risk of acute left ventricular dysfunction in cases of acute vessel occlusion during MV PTCA.

The major problem of long-term follow-up in patients with MV PTCA is the problem of restenosis. As we can show, nearly 50% of the patients had a restenosis of at least one dilated lesion. On the other hand we can show that the incidence of cardiac and myocardial infarction is low (2.2%) because we did further revascularization either by angioplasty (26.2%) or bypass operation (6.5%) during follow-up. In contrast to our findings Reeder [6] and Samson [7] observed a higher incidence of cardiac death [6] and myocardial infarction in patients with incomplete revascularization compared with complete revascularization. Perhaps the lower incidence of revascularization procedures in these studies is the reason for that difference. In accordance with other studies we can show that the incidence of required bypass operations is higher in patients with incomplete revascularization [2,3,6,7]. This finding should encourage interventional cardiologists to try to achieve complete revascularization, although clinical improvement after MV PTCA can be observed during long-term follow-up

Table 3. Cardiac events and clinical follow-up after MV PTCA

Patients (*n*) 229/229; follow-up (mth) 31.2 ± 11.3.

	n	%
Living	223	97.3
Dead		
Noncardiac	3	1.3
Cardiac	3	1.3
Re - PTCA	50	21.8
PTCA other lesion	10	4.4
CABG	15	6.5
AMI	2	0.9
Sum of cardiac events	80	34.9
Angina pectoris		
Improvement	177	79
No change	7	3
Deterioration	38	17

independent of the primarily achieved degree of revascularization.

Clinical implications
MV PTCA can be done without increased risk of acute and long-term ischemic complications with careful patient selection. Patients with MV PTCA show increased risk of restenosis. Therefore, a control angiogram is necessary in order to identify patients with restenosis, and further angioplasty or bypass operation, respectively. In order to reduce the incidence of required bypass operations during follow-up complete revascularization should be the primary therapeutic goal.

References

1. Gruentzig AR, Senning A, Siegenthaler WE (1979) Non-operative dilatation of coronary artery stenosis: Percutaneous transluminal coronary angioplasty. N Engl J Med 301: 61-68.
2. Deligonul U, Vandormael MG, Kern MJ, Zelman R, Galan K, Chaitman BR (1988) Coronary angioplasty: a therapeutic option for symptomatic patients with two and three vessel coronary artery disease. J Am Coll Cardiol 11: 1173-1179.
3. Holmes DR, Vliestra RE, Hammes LN, Reeder GS, Mock MB (1989) Does the disadvantage of incomplete revascularization by coronary angioplasty increase with time? J Am Coll Cardiol 13: 229A.
4. Mabin TA, Holmes DR, Smith HC, Vliestra RE, Reeder GS, Bresnahan JF, Bove AA, Hammes LVN, Elveback LR, Orszulak TA (1985) Follow-up clinical results in patients undergoing transluminal coronary angioplasty. Circulation 71: 754-760.
5. Myler RK, Topol EJ, Shaw RE, Stertzer SH, Clark DA, Fishman J, Murphy MC (1987) Multiple vessel coronary angioplasty: Classification, results, and patterns of restenosis in 494 consecutive patients. Cathet Cardiovasc Diag 13: 1-15.
6. Reeder GS, Holmes DR, Detre K, Costigan T, Kelsey SF (1988) Degree of revascularization in patients with multiple coronary artery disease. A report from the National Heart, Lung, and Blood Institute percutaneous transluminal coronary angioplasty registry. Circulation 77: 638-644.
7. Samson M, Meester HJ, de Feyter PJ, Strauss B, Serruys PW (1990) Successful multiple segment coronary angioplasty: effect of completeness of revascularization in single-vessel multilesions and multivessels. Am Heart J 120: 1-12.
8. Thomas ES, Most AS, Williams DO (1988) Coronary angioplasty in patients with multivessel coronary artery disease: follow-up clinical status. Am Heart J 115: 8-13.
9. Vandormael MG, Chaitman BR, Ischinger T, Aker UT, Harper M, Hernandez J, Deligonul U, Kennedy H (1985) Immediate and short-term benefit of multilesion coronary angioplasty: influence of degree of revascularization. J Am Coll Cardiol 6: 983-991.
10. Gersh BJ, Robertson T (1990) The efficacy of percutaneous transluminal angioplasty (PTCA) in coronary artery disease - Why we need randomized trials. In: EJ Topol, ed. Textbook of Interventional Cardiology. Philadelphia: W.B. Saunders Company, 240-253.
11. Seggewiss H, Fassbender D, Gleichmann U, Vogt J, Mannebach H, Minami K (1991) Perkutane transluminale Koronarangioplastie (PTCA) bei instabiler Angina pectoris: Ergebnisse und Komplikationen unter Berücksichtigung einer neuen Klassifikation. Z Karidol 80: 423-430.
12. Ryan TJ, Faxon DP, Gunnar RM, Kennedy JW, King SB III, Loop FD, Peterson KL, Reeves TJ, Williams DO, Winters WL Jr (1988) Guidelines for percutaneous transluminal coronary angioplasty. A report of the American College of Cardiology/American Heart Association Task

Force on Assessment of Diagnostic and Therapeutic Cardiovascular Procedures (Subcommittee on Percutaneous Transluminal Coronary Angioplasty). Circulation 78: 486–502.

13. Ellis SG, Roubin GS, King SB III, Douglas JS Jr, Shaw RE, Stertzer SH, Myler RK (1988) In-hospital cardiac mortality after acute closure after coronary angioplasty: analysis of risk factors from 8.207 procedures. J Am Coll Cardiol 11: 211–216.

14. Seggewiss H, Fassbender D, Minami K, Schmidt HK, Gleichmann U (in press) Management von Komplikationen bei der PTCA in einer Klinik mit angeschlossener Herzchirurgie. Z Kardiol.

15. Seggewiss H, Fassbender D, Vogt J, Schmidt HK, Volmar J, Mannebach H, Ohlmeier H, Breymann T, Gleichmann U (1990) Beeinflusst die Indikation zur PTCA die Inzidenz der notfallmässigen Bypassoperation? Z Kardiol 79 (Suppl. II): 11.

Index of authors